HOPE

Other Books by Joel Rothschild

*Signals: An Inspiring
Story of Life After Life*

HOPE

A Story of Triumph

Joel Rothschild

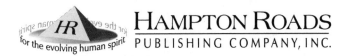

HAMPTON ROADS
PUBLISHING COMPANY, INC.

Cover design by Bartered Graphics
Cover art by Digital Imagery © copyright 2002 PhotoDisc, Inc.

Hampton Roads Publishing Company, Inc.
1125 Stoney Ridge Road
Charlottesville, VA 22902
434-296-2772
fax: 434-296-5096
e-mail: hrpc@hrpub.com
www.hrpub.com

If you are unable to order this book from your local
bookseller, you may order directly from the publisher.
Call 1-800-766-8009, toll-free.

Library of Congress Cataloging-in-Publication Data

Rothschild, Joel, 1957-
   Hope : a story of triumph / Joel Rothschild.
      p. ; cm.
   ISBN 1-57174-353-7 (hard : alk. paper)
   1. Rothschild, Joel, 1957---Health. 2. AIDS
(Disease)--Patients--United States--Biography. 3. Gay men--United
States--Biography. 4. Hope--Psychological aspects.
   [DNLM: 1. Rothschild, Joel, 1957- 2. Acquired Immunodeficiency
Syndrome--psychology--Personal Narratives. 3. Acquired Immunodeficiency
Syndrome--psychology--Popular Works. 4. Survivors-- psychology--Personal
Narratives. 5. Survivors--psychology--Popular Works. 6. Attitude to
Death--Personal Narratives. 7. Attitude to Death-- Popular Works. 8.
Life Change Events--Personal Narratives. 9. Life Change Events--Popular
Works. 10. Pain--psychology--Personal Narratives. 11.
Pain--psychology--Popular Works. 12. Stress,
Psychological--psychology--Personal Narratives. 13. Stress,
Psychological--psychology--Popular Works. WC 503.7 R845h 2002] I.
Title.
   RC606.55.R68 A3 2002
   362.1'9697'920092--dc21

                              2002006960

                    ISBN 1-57174-353-7
                    10 9 8 7 6 5 4 3 2 1
         Printed on acid-free paper in the United States

Dedication

I am blessed to have met many heroes in my life. Each one stands out in my mind, and their common denominator is that they did something that entailed efforts to make this a better planet for others. This book is dedicated to all the named and unnamed heroes that inspired this book. They have all found their way into my life at the most unlikely times and in the most unlikely places, but always with perfect timing. I am certain that the hand of destiny brought them to me. They have all inspired me, and it is my deepest prayer that my life may inspire someone else.

This book is dedicated to my heroes, Barbara Straus-Lodge and Sharon Shaw, whose love continues to sustain me.

And to all my close friends who have given me hope and love.

Table of Contents

Foreword

Heroes, like hope, come in all shapes and sizes. We are inspired by these individuals and often view them as leaders. By virtue of the quality of their actions and the integrity of their intent, they appear to soar. In simply living, they spark a reflection that enables us to sense a bit of our own heroism. It is that common resonance of something so human that is felt here. Hope is so full of potential that it can easily reach through the pages and touch your heart, instilling in you the very hope that you may have felt waning. Joel Rothschild is one of these heroes. His humanity touches our hearts and his story awakens in us the very hope that, at times, we lose sight of.

In *Hope*, you'll read a lot about not just surviving, but thriving; not just about the meaning of life, but of the meaning to life. About acknowledging the commonalities of our human existence in terms of peaks and valleys of emotions, rather than the differences that appear on the surface. You'll read, between the lines, that holding expectations of what the future will bring is a foolish chalice of rose-colored glass. Today, and how we do today, is all we have. Expectations differ from hopes. The fundamentals of hope rest only in believing that there may be a tomorrow. In that most fundamental form, hope requires little structure. It is only when we start romancing the future and coloring its structure with desired rewards, that hope transitions to expectations.

Three years ago, my partner of 18 years died suddenly of a heart attack. The shock and loss were unfathomable, and still, to a great degree, remain so. At that time, Joel's first book, *Signals*, came into my hands. It was like a breath of fresh air. Shortly thereafter, I met Joel and have had the honor to become a friend and doctor to him over the past several years.

You will get to know Joel, the man, in this book. You will see that he is extremely human, vulnerable, and a pit bull of a survivor. Even when his mind thinks he can't make it, his heart and spirit know he can, and he does. Although he may do it more quickly, and certainly with far more creative and articulate skill than many of us, his passionate questioning and seizing of life is described in such a way that we, as readers, can see the process, and in doing so, realize that he is not so different from us.

Regarding Joel, the patient, who continues to survive with AIDS for almost 20 years, I can tell you that what I know of his history is all fact. He is one of the longest-known survivors with HIV infection. He has weathered storms of Kaposi's sarcoma, Pneumocystis pneumonia, and meningitis among other life-threatening opportunistic infections. He has juggled the complications of multiple diagnostic procedures, changing medical regimens, and revolving (some even dying) health care providers, as well as having to shift and repeatedly re-focus insurance issues. And through all that, he is still here.

Most of you reading this will already be believers that attitude and outlook make a difference. To you, this book will be more guiding support. For those of you reading this for the first time who find it difficult to believe that someone might say "having the AIDS virus turned out to be a blessing in disguise," believe me when I say it can be so. Too many times I've been blessed by being a partner in health care for someone diagnosed with a terminal disease. It continually humbles me to watch the emergence of grace and dignity in the most trying of times. In those individuals that for unknown reasons manage to get a few more months or years as a "bonus round," their life outlook often is transformed, and transforming for those around them. I've often heard one say, "if given the choice of being who they would have been without the AIDS virus, or who they are with the AIDS virus, they would definitely choose the latter." One should be very clear that that is a reflection of the clarity and simplicity that are distilled when loss, whether your own or that of ones you love, is near.

I find a fascinating parallel in the tantalizing new area of "psychoneuroimmunology." This is a relatively new field investigating how attitudes, beliefs, and mind-set influence the body and health outcomes. It is remarkable that we are finally getting back to appreciating the exquisitely delicate but important connections between the mind and the immune system. One of the greatest areas of research is focused on the concept of stress. In a most general definition, stress can be physical, mental, emotional, or spiritual angst; it can include more concrete components such as malnutrition or lack of sleep, or simple jet lag. There is a conventional interpretation that "stress" is bad. Stress is not bad. Stress is. It is a component of life and, in fact, it is a necessary component that stimulates us both as whole organisms and, on a cellular level, to respond to some tension in our world. So it's often said that it is not the stress that is unhealthy, but it is one's response to stress that may be so. For it is in the response that we see whether one's coping mechanisms are healthy or unhealthy.

In a way, that is what Joel is saying in this book. He is telling us how he's learned, through feeling and acceptance, to respond to life's inevitable and necessary challenges—but now with a different attitude. And that has made all the difference. He has learned to respond to his stress in a more life-sustaining and health-promoting way. That doesn't change the underlying condition, but it certainly influences the quality of the life he lives. As Elizabeth Kuebler-Ross said on giving advice to survivors of tragedy: "You can tell them that you can't change the direction of the wind. But you can control the setting of the sails." That says it all.

Peter Anton, M. D.

Dr. Peter Anton, M.D., is a graduate of Harvard University. He is one of our nation's most respected HIV research scientists. He is associate professor of medicine at UCLA and director of the UCLA center for HIV research. As a scientist, he works extensively with the National Institute of Health.

Preface

**"Hope and Fear cannot occupy the same space
at the same time. Invite one to stay."**

—Maya Angelou

Now, as I'm writing this book, I'm keenly aware that this time is my bonus round.

It has been a long road, and today, I'm one of the longest-living AIDS survivors. I've already outlived two of my doctors' predictions of imminent death. I've even outlived three of my doctors. I have lived with full-blown AIDS for most of my adult life. So, it's possible I'll have passed on by the time you are reading my words. Whether or not I am alive doesn't diminish the possibilities this book contains for you.

During the time I've lived with AIDS more than twenty million people have died from it. That's almost the entire population of New York and Los Angeles combined. I'm constantly asked how I've survived while millions perished. The answer is contained within these pages. But this is not a book about merely surviving; it's about thriving. This is not a book about dying; it's about living.

The events I've chronicled within these pages are deeply personal experiences. You'll come to know me as you read this book. I am grateful knowing that you will be reading my words. You are adding meaning to my existence, and it is my intention to add meaning to yours.

In many ways, we may be different, and in many ways, we are the same. We will both experience many of the same joys in life and will share some of the same agonies. The different ways we suffer are not important. It is what we glean from that suffering that counts. Please try to relate to me as a human being rather than a gay man with AIDS. Today, I'm able to go through months of extreme physical pain with profound acceptance and peace. I've even found purpose and meaning in the suffering. It's not always been this way. After a journey filled with extraordinary transitions, I'm living a life without fear. I now see that I've been blessed by AIDS. I've accepted the circumstances of my life and used both the good and the bad as catalysts for propelling me forward on a path to truly living.

There are two Joel Rothschilds: one that experienced life before AIDS and one that was dramatically changed by AIDS. Humbling and momentous, this disease changed my life in a way that nothing else could ever have done. I could never have predicted my own experiences with loss. Hope transformed trauma into a new beginning. Sometimes, the most complicated problems in our lives have the simplest answer, and the most frightening situations help us return to what's really important in life. We all have the ability to be survivors. Often we are simply unaware of the tools we already possess. The power to transcend loss lies within all of us.

If you are suffering right now, know this; it will pass. Our spirits are amazingly resilient. Time alone can soften pain and loss and replace it with a warm glow. Nothing lasts forever, not even joy and bliss. We will all experience highs and lows in this life, and at some point, our lives as we have come to know them will end. Therefore, it seems best to live life on its own terms, with acceptance, peace, and hope.

When I look back on my life, I realize that AIDS propelled me to a place of peace and joy. It challenged me to find new meaning in my life, to become a more compassionate person. I now realize that pain and loss have been essential to the growth in my life. I have become a better person from suffering, and I know you too can learn from my losses.

So many people learn only by beating their heads against a wall. I know this is true because I used to do it, too. Within these pages there lies an opportunity for you to benefit from my struggles. You can transcend pain and suffering, and this may become your epiphany as well. You can come to enjoy life in ways you never thought possible, and your challenges will become a source of strength. Here is the opportunity to gain clarity about your life and to free yourself from worry and grief.

One good thing about living with a fatal disease is that you don't get caught up in the illusion that you have time to waste. I pray you realize this, and that you discover each day of life is your bonus round. Not one day of our life is to be wasted. Don't wait for a brush with death or a terminal illness to learn this lesson. That's the point of my writing this book for you.

Chapter 1

April 22, 1986:

The First Long Night—Fear

**"It is when the well's dry, that
we know the worth of the water."**

—Benjamin Franklin

Every day of life is a gift. I have noticed that
in the rush of everyday living, most people
overlook the precious nature of our very existence. One of the remarkable advantages of
surviving a plane crash or any brush with death
is that one assumes a more profound appreciation for every moment of life. People who survived the holocaust or any intense disaster
recognize the terms and conditions that a second chance at life can contain. Our lease on life
is renewed and changed. Passion and purpose
are made self-evident to those of us who value
time. As our denial of death is stripped away,
we gain a deeper appreciation for the richness
that is every moment of life. The simple act of

acknowledging our mortality allows us to embrace and savor life.

It is natural not to want to feel the pain of a loss. But there is no escape. Drugs, drinking, eating, gambling, sex, shopping, money, work, and any other form of suppression can only temporarily numb the pain. They cannot free you from it. The only way out of pain is to go directly though it. It is when we push it away that it will haunt us.

I'm sorry that some of what I have to share may not be comfortable to hear. I need to talk to you about death and loss for you to expand your consciousness. At some point in life, we all will experience death. Perhaps we will lose a parent, sibling, or friend. Some of us may even experience the agonizing loss of a child or spouse. We live our lives thinking this won't happen to us. When it does, these losses can send anyone reeling into a depression. But, they can also be catalysts to propel us into the light.

Pain and loss are not all bad. With the passing of time, my losses have had a life-affirming effect. Suffering led to questions about what is going on around and within me. Without those questions there would have been no answers. Through loss, life becomes a precious opportunity for development and enlightenment. It is the challenges in life that force us to examine the nature of our existence. Suffering forces us to change and can guide us to our deepest truth. Within this book is an opportunity for you to learn without suffering and a chance to create joy in every moment of your life.

Parts of this book may be off-putting to read. Even now, at the onset of our journey, I am asking that you consider the fact that someday you will die. Even if you don't have AIDS or a terminal illness, your death is coming, as is my own. We just don't know the date and time. It is a significant achievement to accept that our time here will expire. Perhaps you will put your denial aside as I try my best to tell you about the day I first heard my death sentence. Let me convey to you what it feels like to be given one. The fear and sadness are unimaginable. It is important that you know what it feels like to be faced with your own mortality. By embracing your own inevitable passing you will become free to live your life to the fullest. The moment that you accept and realize your mortality you will become stronger than you have ever imagined. It was disease that helped me find my inner strength. Rather than seeing myself as a victim, I came to see myself as a survivor. I wasn't in denial. I always knew the odds were stacked against me; however, when I faced my mortality, I became stronger.

I have been an athlete my entire life. From swimming to weight training, I love working out. By my early twenties, I was a competitive athlete, and bodybuilding had become an essential part of my life. I found extreme pleasure in testing my physical limits. For more than a decade, I measured my health by my daily workouts. I was in prime shape and always healthy.

During the first months of 1986, I had been training regularly, but my strength was failing. I attributed the decrease in strength to my approaching thirtieth birthday. I became determined to work out even harder. I increased my fourteen-hour-a week regimen into a challenging twenty hours. At one hundred and sixty pounds, I was bench-pressing more than three hundred and fifty pounds. Naturally, I thought I was in good health. My grandparents had lived into their nineties. I assumed I had fifty or sixty good years ahead. I had hoped to die in my sleep as a very old person who had lived a rich and fulfilling life.

In March, I noticed some small bumps around my neck, under the skin's surface. I thought they were ingrown hairs and ignored

them. One day, while training, I saw a derma-
tologist acquaintance. In the middle of my
workout, I decided to ask him about the
bumps. He felt them and strongly suggested I
go see my regular doctor.

I ignored his suggestion to see Dr. Roth, who
had been my physician for several years. As the
next few weeks passed, working out became
increasingly difficult. Finally, I was short of
breath climbing the stairwell up to the weight
room. I assumed I was just tired. Perhaps I
needed a few days to recover. I decided to take
the next three days off and go to the beach. By
the third day, I was running a low-grade fever. I
simply attributed this to too much sun. The
next night, I woke up at four A.M. drenched in
sweat. My sheets were as soaked as if they had
just come out of the washing machine. I got up,
turned my thermostat down to sixty degrees
and lay on top of my comforter. After an hour,
I could tell the room was cold, but I was still
sweating and the comforter was drenched. My
temperature was only slightly higher than normal, but I suspected something was terribly
wrong. I waited until morning and telephoned
Dr. Roth.

By the time I met with Dr. Roth, my fever
had soared to 103.5 degrees. Dr. Roth took

some x-rays, blood tests, and a lung-function test. He told me that the bumps were swollen lymph nodes and that I had a very low-level lung function. He wanted to rush me to Saint John's Hospital in an ambulance. I must have been in denial about the seriousness of my condition because I remember I asked why I couldn't drive the few miles myself. Yet, I felt so weak. I didn't argue with him and acquiesced. I was more embarrassed about being wheeled out of the building on a gurney than I was concerned about having AIDS.

When we arrived at the hospital I refused to let anyone assist me; I attempted to walk on my own. A small, frail nurse brought me a wheel chair. I was so dizzy, I fell into the wheel chair. The nurse wheeled me into the huge stainless steel elevator that would carry us to the third floor. Before we entered the room, the nurse put on gloves and a mask, which seemed odd, as if I had been labeled "contaminated." The thought made me angry and defensive.

As I entered the room my head was spinning; all I wanted to do was lie down. The nurse summoned two orderlies to help me into the tiny bed. I was indignant and didn't want to be lifted from the chair. I uttered something rude about the small size of the bed. The nurse snapped back that its size was the least of my worries. I noticed I was in a white room with only one bed. I was in quarantine. I was extremely weak and felt disassociated from my surroundings and myself. After they put me into the bed, they enclosed me in a plastic tent that covered the bed. I was so out of sorts that I didn't feel the nurse start the intravenous drip. I fell asleep as she gently lifted my head to put an oxygen mask over my face.

I awoke a few hours later gasping for air. My lungs were filled with fluid, and I was desperately trying to breathe. Soon, I was on several more intravenous medications in the hopes of curtailing the infection and preventing further assaults on my now-fragile immune system. Pain extended from my lungs and upper respiratory tract all the way down into my lower back. I was vacillating between feeling the sharp pain and experiencing the numbing effect of the painkillers they gave me.

The next day, Dr. Roth came to check on me. My first question was about my diagnosis. He told me I had pneumonia. For a moment I felt relieved. Then he told me I had full-blown AIDS. The words didn't register at first. I went into emotional shock. I listened as he explained the test results and the situation I was facing.

Towards the end of his explanation, I asked if I was going to die. His answer was nervous, short, and filled with fear. He didn't look at me.

Dr. Roth explained normal T-cell counts are between six hundred and two thousand, but because my immune system was already ravaged, mine were dangerously less than one hundred. In spite of the severity of the situation, he thought I was strong enough to make it through this infection. Before I could take comfort in his prognosis, he uttered, "I think you'll have one year of decent health; beyond that, there are no promises or guarantees. The life expectancy for anyone in your condition is under one year."

Those few words were violent and powerful. A hot flash of nervous energy exploded and ricocheted through every cell of my body. My heart began to pound, and I felt its heavy beating in my chest. My nerves crawled like bugs through my skin. My thoughts raced. I felt suicidal, scared, and sad, at the same time. I wanted to run, scream, do something, but was too weak to stand. Time stood still. Fear washed over me.

Dr. Roth was still talking about my immediate medical prognosis, but I didn't hear another word. I was immobilized by fear. Eventually, he left me alone. After a few moments of stunned silence, tears began to flow from my eyes. I sank into an overwhelming and all-consuming depression. This was the first time in my life I recognized my own mortality, and I felt helpless. Death was on its way much sooner than I had ever dreamt. My life would never be the same. In a few moments I had lost everything I had ever known. AIDS had changed everything.

After what seemed like hours of convulsive sobbing and agonizing images of sickness and death flashing through my head, a nurse entered the room to change one of my intravenous bags. She was kind and gentle with me, but nothing anyone could say could comfort me. Not wanting to cry in front of her, I held back my tears until she left the room. Alone again, I cried until I drifted off into a fitful sleep.

I was awakened by a long-forgotten memory. I began to have something between déjà vu and a flashback. I was wide awake. The event I recalled had actually happened but it seemed like a vivid dream. I was reliving a moment from 1982 when I was visiting my friend Chris in Atlanta's Piedmont Hospital. He was nineteen, I was twenty-six at the time. My flashback was like a play within a play. I remembered Chris's little white isolation room; it was nearly identical to mine. I was alone with him in his room. I took off my mask and gloves. I had no way of knowing the gravity of the situation or what was to become of Chris. At the time, we didn't know what AIDS was. It had just surfaced on the medical scene and Chris would be the first person I would know with the virus. The disease didn't even have a name yet. As we talked, Chris kept attempting to shift the conversation to death. He would say things like "I'm not afraid to die" and "I'm ready to go."

I wondered if he was coherent. There was an unfamiliar, peaceful, tranquil feeling in Chris's room. He had always been soft spoken and on this visit he was particularly calm. I remember thinking that maybe he was right and perhaps he was really going to die.

It didn't register then, but now I know he had been trying to say good-bye to me. I kept offering him inane, idle conversation. I never said good-bye. Chris died the next day.

It now hit me that Chris's death was the closest I had ever come to experiencing death myself. Now, I wasn't only remembering his sense of knowing and acceptance; I was reliving it with him. I reflected on the tranquillity I felt with him. Strangely, my memories of Chris calmed me. Even so, I did not want to die. It was not death I feared; it was missing life. There were so many things I'd yet to experience. There were books I wanted to read, places to see, friends I would miss. I wanted to live at least until my thirtieth birthday.

During that first night in quarantine, I remembered another friend who had died in 1985 from the same kind of lung infection I was now fighting. It seemed logical that if both friends died from pneumonia, then surely I would follow the same path. It would have been easy to surrender to those thoughts of dread. For a short time I did and called my parents in Miami to tell them I was dying. We cried together over the phone.

After days of relentless tears, I finally looked inside myself. I found tiny molecules of hope. I knew I didn't want to surrender to my illness. I began to realize this battle would have to be waged on several levels, not just the physical. I lay in quarantine losing my last shreds of vanity. My single concern was staying alive. I thought there must be a level of consciousness I could reach to survive any great challenge. People who make it to the top of Mount Everest, win Olympic gold medals, or survive extreme physical challenges must have mastered their thought processes. They have learned to eliminate self-sabotage. I actually began forcing myself to think positively about surviving. I used every once of courage I could muster to be optimistic.

Physically, I struggled to focus on simple things like movement, eating, and breathing. It was not easy but I forced myself to sit upright, or get out of bed and walk around the room. When it was mealtime, I asked for extra portions and struggled to eat them in the belief that the extra food would fuel my strength. In those moments when my lungs felt clear I would cherish the long, deep breaths I could take. Instead of thinking about the time I was losing to my illness, I constantly thought about the possibility of surviving. I pushed myself to think about things in life I enjoyed. I clung to hope despite my circumstances. I hoped to walk out of Saint John's Hospital and once again join the living. I promised myself I would never take life for granted again. I have often thought about the defining moments in my life. I realize now that those tiny molecules of hope became the foundation for my survival.

At the time, Robert Cohen, Tony Hamilton, Kelly Cole, and Mark Simon were my closest friends. We were like a family. I never had a brother so knowing Robert was like having one. I had met him in Hebrew School when we both were thirteen. We had enjoyed a close friendship ever since junior high. Robert and I met Tony when we were in college in 1976, and almost from the moment we met we became inseparable. Our time together was spent mostly laughing. People would often refer to us as either The Three Musketeers or The Three Stooges. Tony was an actor, and on the set of a movie he met Kelly. Kelly was the son of Nat King Cole. The two of them dated for a short time in 1982. Kelly effortlessly wove his way into our lives. During 1984 I had met and dated Mark Simon. He had a deep love for life and a wonderful sense of humor. I admired those traits in Mark, and he rounded out our little clan. My friends could lift my spirits in the bleakest of times, but by 1986 all my friends were HIV positive. It was a scary time for people who were HIV positive and healthy to see people develop full-blown AIDS. Always the most serious, I had been the emotional anchor of the group. I was deeply concerned about their reaction and didn't want to be a burden for them. However, I finally mustered the courage to call. The four of them immediately came to the hospital.

They were adamant that I could survive. Kelly was a natural entertainer. He would spend hours in my room telling stories about celebrities he had known from his childhood. Kelly, Mark, and Tony would break the hospital rules by bringing in fresh flowers and taking turns sitting by my side throughout the night. One of them stayed with me continuously from that point on. When we were together, I felt stronger than when I was alone.

When I was finally released from the hospital, my life did not return to normal. I was nauseous all the time. Expending the slightest effort fatigued me. I was constantly run down. My way of living had been thrown into a tailspin. I could only live with the malaise of my lingering symptoms by accepting them as a respite from the hospital experience. I slept a lot, believing I was gaining strength by allowing my body the rest it needed. At times, the fatigue was so severe that my body felt weighed down with lead. I had to make many adjustments just to live a semi-normal life. It wasn't easy. There were times I couldn't talk or even eat. On those days I would lie in bed fighting the nausea and only get up to use the bathroom. I looked pale and wasted. Despite my circumstance I was steadfast in my determination to survive. I forced myself to be as active as possible and stay hopeful.

Instead of a death sentence, the lung infection became the first of several key turning points. A tiny voice inside me wasn't ready to let me surrender. It kept saying, "NO. YOU WILL SURVIVE AND YOU WILL LIVE." Perhaps it was the voice of denial, or perhaps it was the beginning of a spiritual shift. Either way, I made an internal choice to hold on. This was the classic moment for a "flight or fight" reaction; I chose to fight. I didn't know what I was fighting for or the source of my inner strength, and under the circumstances it would have been rational to relinquish any optimism. But I couldn't ignore the tiny voice, despite my fear.

Chapter 2

An Act of Kindness

"You cannot do a kindness too soon, for you never know how soon it will be too late."

—Ralph Waldo Emerson

In the months that followed my stay at Saint Johns Hospital, I was extremely weak. One day, I began to notice a few bruises on my body. I hadn't sustained any injuries and I couldn't figure out where they came from. They were dark and disfiguring and multiplied as time passed. I couldn't figure out why I was getting these bruises. I ignored them for several weeks. Then, I started to have frequent nosebleeds, my gums began to bleed, and the bleeding occurred at the most inopportune times. This became more and more frequent, lasted longer, and became nearly impossible to stop.

One day while driving, I had a nosebleed more severe than usual and noted the blood was thin and watery. This nosebleed lasted more than two hours. It could not be ignored, and finally I went to see my doctor. After we did blood tests, he said he was surprised I was still walking. Normally, platelets number in the hundreds of thousands (from 130,000 to 400,000/mm[3]; less than fifty thousand is cause for concern; less than ten thousand is life threatening. My platelet count hovered at eleven thousand: This condition is known as idiopathic thrombocytopenic purpura (ITP for short). It's a form of an autoimmune illness that results in the destruction of blood platelets. When the platelet count becomes exceedingly low it can cause spontaneous bleeding. Platelet counts under ten thousand can lead to hemorrhaging in the brain and result in death.

My body was having this autoimmune response due to the HIV virus. It was turning on itself and shutting down the production of normal cells essential for healthy living. Dr. Roth suggested rushing me to an operating room to remove my spleen. The operation would release stored platelets from my spleen into my body. He suggested the surgery was the best way to go.

At the time, almost nothing about AIDS was known for certain. Every procedure was marked with uncertainty and a lack of substantial data. We didn't have the luxury of the Internet and its research possibilities. I questioned Dr. Roth about alternatives to surgery. He told me that Elizabeth Taylor's fledgling organization, the American Foundation for AIDS Research (amfAR), had just produced the first AIDS treatment guide in the world. It might have some alternative information regarding ITP treatment. As luck would have it, the only drug study in the world was being conducted in my backyard, at Los Angeles County/ USC Medical Center in Los Angeles. It was an experimental treatment. I didn't want surgery, so I would attempt to qualify for that study.

The experimental study entailed taking sixteen azidothymidine (AZT) pills a day combined with massive IV infusions of gamma globulin every week. I hoped to qualify for the study because I had heard about this new experimental drug, AZT. The idea of getting any treatment for my AIDS seemed a positive step. This was an ideal opportunity to treat the ITP and AIDS at the same time.

I went to the county hospital AIDS clinic the next day to sign up for the study. The clinic was the most horrific place I'd ever seen. The hospital was run down and dilapidated. The county hospital was the last refuge for the sick and indigent. The drug study for ITP was done at 5p21—the designated AIDS ward. The ward had been relegated to the most dank, dismal region of the hospital and resembled a concentration camp. People were milling about struggling to get into studies. For many, these studies were their last chance for hope. Adding to everyone's frustration and desperation was the fact that most of the studies were conducted as double-blind studies, which meant that even if someone was "lucky" enough to have just the right blood counts to qualify, there was still a fifty-fifty chance of receiving a placebo rather than the actual, potentially life-saving drug. Half of these human guinea pigs would come to the clinic for months, participate in the hope of gaining improvement, only to find that they had not received any treatment and then eventually die.

This seemed an unusually cruel procedure to me. People were dying every day. Many had visible opportunistic infections, like Kaposi's sarcoma spreading over their bodies or Molluscum, an AIDS-related wart, growing on their faces. Others were wasting away from the never-ending onslaught of unseen opportunistic infections that descended upon people whose immune systems were devastated.

At the clinic, they were doing their best to treat active infections. At the same time, they were conducting studies for then-untreatable life-threatening opportunistic infections. The feeling in the clinic halls was like that on a sinking ship, with everyone clamoring to escape, but there weren't enough life rafts, and people were drowning.

Death in the dark ages of AIDS was a great equalizer. The rich were in the same sinking boat as the destitute. People of all races and backgrounds were forced together by desperate circumstances. The appearance of people with jaundiced skin and bruised and haggard bodies was like a horror movie. But this was real.

The doctors and nurses were helpless. There were limited resources and too many sick people. Some doctors and nurses responded by disconnecting from it all: they treated their patients like objects. AIDS was taking its toll on them as well; they became distant and cold. It was a terrible time for everybody.

Soon, I learned that a spinal tap was required for me to be on the study. Mine was performed in a tiny, converted broom closet. It had two small folding doors at each end and no windows and was set in the middle of two open hallways. I was lucky and got on the study. I found out from another patient that you could open and taste your AZT pills. You would know you were not on a placebo if the taste was bitter. I was getting the real drug.

When I received my weekly IV treatments, I would often leave the clinic with my arms covered in bruises due to the inexperience of the nurses who administered the drips. I dreaded the nurses almost as much as going to the clinic itself. In 5p21 there were no amenities, no time for kindness, and not enough time to dig graves.

This was not a place for friendships, and most people kept their distance. But I couldn't help myself, I befriended a young couple—a twenty-year-old named Brian, who would roar up on a motorcycle with his nineteen-year-old girlfriend, Jean. I met them on my second week at the clinic. She was Italian and strikingly beautiful with long, black hair and bright blue eyes. He was Jewish, low key and normal looking. They were both from Riverside and had been dating since high school. She had AIDS-related lymphoma, and it was attacking her brain. She was on an experimental chemotherapy that also required IV infusions. We were often scheduled at the same time.

We endured our three-hour infusions, which were even more uncomfortable because they were done in a large, open hallway that doubled as the patient waiting room.

Whenever the three of us could, we sat together for conversation and support. During one of our conversations, I asked Brian if he was HIV positive. He told me that in high school, Jean had done volunteer work with underprivileged children in Compton. In her sophomore year, she was assaulted and raped by gang members. At sixteen, she contracted the AIDS virus from the rape and had unsuspectingly passed it on to him.

Despite the tragedy of their circumstances they remained upbeat and visibly in love. He appeared totally devoted to her. They seemed like two small-town kids in a movie, falling in love for the first time. They held hands and he constantly told her how beautiful she was. For a time, their love even brightened the dismal confines of 5p21.

I remember everything at the clinic as gray. The walls were gray, people were gray, the mood was always gray. It seemed amazing to see the brilliance of Jean and Brian's love in such gray surroundings. I wondered if they were unaware of the gravity of what they were facing. Regardless, I was grateful for them as they helped make things bearable for me. As the weeks passed, Jean began to lose her hair from the treatments, and she lost weight. Later, she became despondent. I wondered how she could tolerate the motorcycle ride home with the nausea from the infusion. In time, she looked thin, barren, and worse, until finally he was practically carrying her frail body in for her treatments. All the while, Brian attended to her as if she was the most beautiful woman in the world and he was the luckiest guy to be with her.

I missed seeing them for a couple of weeks and finally asked one of our regular nurses if she had seen them lately. Without looking up from what she was doing and without providing any details she simply said, "Jean died." Even now, fifteen years later, as I think of them I feel the same sadness of that moment in 5p21.

At 5p21, making friends could impose the steep price on you of feeling more pain. Yet, I couldn't close myself off emotionally from the people who were sharing my suffering. Another person I met during the treatment, was a small eighty-six-year-old woman named Eleanor. She would clutch her little, black 1940s-style vinyl purse, had immaculately coifed blue-gray hair, and always wore a starched Sunday-best dress. She looked as if she had just arrived from church.

Eleanor was there with her son, whom she

drove from Long Beach for his weekly treatments. They had no other family, and there was no one there to help her. During our first few conversations, her son was in a private room, and I never met him. I formed a mental picture of what I imagined him to look like, figuring him to be in his mid-forties.

When I finally met him, I was shocked to see that he was actually in his late sixties. He looked almost as old as his mother. He looked as out of place in the clinic as his mother did. It seemed odd to think of an older man with AIDS. I hadn't considered AIDS as being multi-generational.

After a few more weeks, he too died, and I never saw Eleanor again. I often thought about her, alone, burying her only child. For weeks after Jean and then Eleanor's son had died, I sat alone in the ward with the other patients, not looking at anyone, not speaking to anyone, head down, wishing I was anywhere but 5p21. Alone, I found the surroundings even more depressing. There was no privacy, no comfort, no security. The hospital was like a tomb with bad fluorescent lighting. The walls and floors were concrete, dirty, and demoralizing. I understood firsthand the reason for the emotional barrier people built up around themselves in

5p21. If you got close to someone and they died, you experienced the grief of losing a new friend coupled with the chilling reminder of your own desperate situation and looming mortality. A part of me tried to put up walls and not talk to anybody again, but I guess it wasn't in my nature.

When I finally shook myself out of my self-imposed isolation, I became determined again to befriend as many people as possible. I made an effort to greet, and compliment, and smile at everyone I could. I would find anything positive, pleasant, or kind to say to the other patients or the staff. Whenever possible, I would practice the smallest acts of kindness or generosity even with the sickest or most disfigured people; I struggled to not look away and to find anything positive to say to them, no matter how minor. To comment on a haircut, a new pair of shoes, the weather, it didn't really matter, I would find something nice to say.

Also, I listened to the other patients in 5p21. Everyone was desperate to be heard. Possibly it was a last attempt to be remembered. I listened out of genuine interest and was rewarded by hearing wisdom. It was then that I became aware of the unique qualities that kept some people alive beyond medical predictions.

These people held an unshakable belief that they would overcome their disease, and they almost always lived substantially longer than those who did not. I witnessed people finding new meaning in times of mortal danger.

I took those lessons to heart and began to search for ways to reinvent myself and give new meaning to my life. I became involved in political activism to change the FDA's antiquated system of testing new drugs. I was learning to put into practice the profound optimism I saw extending other people's lives. Years later a doctor would confirm what I learned in 5p21. He told me that no disease in the history of humanity has ever been one hundred percent fatal . . . maybe ninety-nine percent, but never one hundred. In the face of even the deadliest diseases, a few people have always survived. The black plague, the most virulent cancers, and even the Ebola virus all had survivors. I believe these survivors were all positively altered by their circumstances. I was becoming determined to survive.

The process of being transformed into an emotionally healthier person began when I became determined to join that small percentage of survivors. Soon my trips to the clinic became marked by paradox. I was feeling better and stronger, while almost everyone around me was getting worse. I was very lucky, and my body was responding to the treatments.

One day, in the midst of all the insanity of 5p21 and my own fears, I was stopped in my tracks by the tiny voice inside my head, this time it cried out; "THIS IS IT . . . you might have one year or one day, but it's definitely time to stop waiting for life to happen and start living as if each day is your last."

I began reassessing and redefining everything about who I was and what I stood for. I learned to stand on my own and to take good care of myself. I was learning to fight for my life and not to squander my time by living under a cloud of impending doom. I realized that life is seldom fair, and we don't always get what we think we deserve. Sometimes, bad things do happen to unsuspecting good people. Often, that's just the way life goes.

However, we have choices in how we interpret our circumstances and how we react to them. I believe that we are capable of ascending to a level of diplomacy and acceptance with life. The difference is you can either battle, hammer, and fight, or you can mediate.

Diplomacy is one of the loftiest things we can do with our communication. Since we are able to attain peace with our enemies, on whom better to apply this skill than ourselves?

The infusions had brought my platelet count up to thirty-eight thousand, and I was out of immediate danger. The AZT seemed to be keeping the virus in check and my other blood counts were getting progressively better. For a few months, I felt almost normal.

Then one night I planned a small dinner party for Mark's birthday. My friends and I went shopping to buy him a gift. After an hour of walking around, I felt a pounding in my head and ringing in my ears. After another hour, it got so bad I had to walk back to the car. Before we got to the escalator, I collapsed and blacked out. Tony and Kelly carried me to Robert's car and drove me to the USC emergency room.

At the emergency room, we learned that I had a side effect from the high level of AZT. My body repressed production of normal red blood cells to a near fatal level. The drugs had rapidly wiped out my hemoglobin count. Hemoglobin transports oxygen to vital areas of the body, and a normal value of hemoglobin is twelve to fifteen. I was below five, and my blood was nearly depleted of hemoglobin. That day I was stabilized after receiving whole blood by transfusion for six hours.

Now I faced a new fear, that I would be dropped from the study due to the rigorous restrictions regarding side effects. I knew if I was dropped, I would have no way of receiving the potentially life-saving experimental drugs.

My fears were realized the following week when I was unceremoniously dropped from the study. I now understood the desperation of many of patients at the clinic. The thought even crossed my mind that I would be willing to commit armed robbery to get the drugs I needed to stay alive. I talked with Tony and Mark about stealing drugs. Instead of responding in shock, they were both open to the idea. We had a frank discussion about the details and the method of our "break-in" to the 5p21 pharmacy. Of course, we didn't have the guts for it. We were surprised, however, that we never heard of anyone else taking those drastic steps.

In the early days of the AIDS pandemic, there were a handful of unsung heroes. These heroes were doctors willing to put their medical licenses on the line in the hopes of saving lives. These doctors would hoard drugs originally intended for patients on a study who then died. The doctors would share these surplus drugs with patients who desperately needed them but who didn't qualify to receive them under the stringent requirements.

As fate would have it I was assigned to one of these heroic renegades. He asked me not to tell anyone he was providing me with the drugs. He lowered my dosage to a tolerable level. He kept me on AZT even though I was officially off the study. I remained stable during the next year and a half. The drug did its job and kept me alive long enough to receive the next round of experimental drugs. In the midst of the madness of 5p21, a doctor who didn't know me, who could have lost everything, followed his heart and saved my life.

We may never know what springs from our acts of kindness. The gift we give to others and the world when we act selflessly is an unseen ripple that extends through time. No matter how small, our individual acts of bravery and kindness can have an effect on the whole of humanity.

This book is proof of that fact. You would not be holding it in your hands if that doctor hadn't given me the gift of his kindness fifteen years ago. That act of kindness years ago allowed you and me to converge in this moment.

Chapter 3

Now Is the Moment

"Dost thou love life? Then do not squander time, for that's the stuff life is made of."

—Benjamin Franklin

In the two years that followed, I had six hospitalizations for different opportunistic infections. Even when I was not in the hospital there were many days I couldn't leave my bed. Other times, I would spend a day's worth of energy just showering, getting dressed, and eating. Often, it took all my strength to take a short walk. I set many small, reachable goals to carry me through these bad days. Whenever possible, I pushed myself to take short walks, which sometimes became longer walks. I envisioned myself in good health. My vision of surviving would not be enough to keep me alive. I put vision into action and made it my intention to survive. I made efforts to stay active every day despite how I felt. On some days it took all the stamina I had to get out of bed, but I did it anyway.

My pilgrimage to healing continued with practical steps. I replaced bodybuilding with cardiovascular training. It was my way of countering the disease and regaining some control over my body. I pushed myself to train. I told myself, "I can do this, and I will get stronger." Cardiovascular fitness kept me feeling healthier. Perhaps it's because of the endorphin release or the extra oxygen that gets pumped through the body, but I always felt better after doing it. I gave up alcohol and coffee. I drank more water and ate healthier. I ate fresh fruits, vegetables, fish, and nuts. I sought laughter in the company of friends. I refused to see sad or violent movies; I watched only comedies. I made it a point to not be alone when I was feeling either sad or angry.

Most important, I learned to live life in the moment, and I allowed myself time to rest. I stopped thinking about things outside my immediate control. I slowed down the pace of my life, emotionally and physically. I learned to be fully present in each individual moment of my life. I took up daily meditation and prayer. I continued by making the simple acts of sleeping and eating top priorities. I would not address any issue if I had not slept or eaten sufficiently first. I learned to be more grateful, to take comfort in the things millions of people can only dream about, things I had always taken for granted: a well-stocked refrigerator; a soft warm bed; clean, drinkable running water; a long hot shower. Tiny bits of hope, combined with the simplest actions, produced epic healing results.

I was learning to become an optimist. When confronted with negative emotions, I noticed my initial failure to slow down long enough to recognize and neutralize these destructive thoughts. Then I started to slow down and become self-observant. I stayed focused on the positive, and lived in the present. I became aware of my internal dialogue. Awareness is half the battle. Slowing down helped lessen my stress level so I could catch and isolate my negativity. I found great strength in stillness.

One can attain a new dimension of consciousness by slowing down and focusing on the present. We all have an internal dialogue that happens so quickly and spontaneously most of us are not even aware it. When you begin to know the dialogue exists, you can begin healing by stopping the parts of the dialogue that are subliminally self-sabotaging. I could not afford the luxury of any internal negativity. It is truly a decadent luxury to engage in such acts of self-destruction. If you think your life will last forever, then maybe you can waste your time in pessimism and negativity. But no one lives forever. Time is precious.

Negative feelings and judgments, such as anger, envy, guilt, fear, worry, and resentment, must be understood and released, or they will poison you. They will drain you of the vital energy needed to sustain your life. I made it a habit to check in on my emotional status. I began by asking myself; what's going on inside me at this moment? I made every effort to change fearful emotional and mental patterns. There is a reward when you stop judging and forgive. That reward is inner peace.

My priorities totally changed, being in a battle for survival. In my time of crisis, I was forced to put first things first and make every effort to take proper care of myself. At first this seemed overwhelming, but the price for not doing it was the potential to spiral downward into a worsening condition. We can only become fully alive here and now by staying present. The seeds of peace and acceptance are within each one of us, and they are ready for cultivation.

We are all too amply endowed with the ability to create additional pain for ourselves by engaging in the fantasy of "What if" thinking. If we leave our present moment and do this, we risk opening a Pandora's box of imaginary misery and releasing it into an already difficult experience. The results can be more devastating and destructive than the original problem. Psychological conditions like fear, anxiety, and tension are divorced from actual physical pain. The largest part of human pain is unnecessary and self-created. The more you leave the present moment and worry about projected pain, the more you will suffer.

The more you are able to accept your present moment, the more you are free from suffering. By staying present and staying conscious, you can guard against creating additional discomfort. Feelings such as nervousness and dread are lessened by staying in the moment. Even though it is impossible for anyone to remain completely in the moment all the time, with practice we can develop the skills to remain in the present more often than not. By developing these skills we will lead a healthier life. The key to this ability lies in slowing down and becoming self-observant. You must learn to recognize your own internal dialogues before you can effectively change them. Often that awareness itself is enough to diminish them.

By March of 1989 my dear friend Robert's health had worsened. We always seemed to be accompanying each other on our visits to doctors. Yet, we considered ourselves lucky to be alive and on a variety of experimental drugs. We were physically weaker and also being challenged emotionally. He was less optimistic than I. AIDS seemed to be everywhere in our community, and almost weekly someone we knew died; a clerk in a store, a bank teller, or the partner of an acquaintance. We were always being invited to memorial services. Local mortuaries, estate planners, viatacals (companies that specialize in purchasing life insurance from the terminally ill) and home health-care companies were placing daily ads in the local gay newspapers, competing for the growing business of sickness and death. I joined a weekly AIDS support group with twenty-seven members in 1986. By December of 1989, only two people in the group remained alive. When we stopped seeing someone around town we were never certain if he had died or moved away. We were living amid a modern-day holocaust, in which people were constantly slipping away. I did not want anyone to be forgotten. I wanted to remember as many people as I could. I began writing the word "dead" in red ink across the names of victims in my phone book. By the end of 1990, thirty-seven souls had been memorialized by my red ink.

I felt extremely blessed having my four friends alive. We went to the theater or movies as often as possible. I loved to cook, and we would get together at my place once or twice a week. After dinner, we always played cards. We enjoyed each other's company and would get lost in conversations about our lives, the arts, politics, and love. On those nights, we were able to smile, laugh, and somehow forget about AIDS. Together we were stronger than alone and were able to keep our spirits up. We were all fighting to maintain some sense of normalcy and hope in our lives.

As that year progressed, Robert's health failed quickly. He seemed to encounter one opportunistic infection after another in a continual assault on his immune system. Robert had always been my closest friend, and I worried that he might die. I decided to spend as much time as possible with Robert. I saw how easily life can be snatched away. I realized I should share my love in the living years by making certain that I told him everything I ever wanted to. We talked often about the fun we had as teenagers, reminisced about silly things from our past: going to discos at age fifteen with fake IDs; reading about our high school nemesis, a bully named Steve, who got arrested for soliciting a prostitute; our first motorcycle ride; and thousands of other memories. When we talked about our personal history we would break into uncontrollable laughter. We laughed so hard it hurt. I thanked Robert often for the way he helped shape my life.

Robert's health worsened that year. It seemed obvious he would soon die. He was always coughing; he had gotten terribly gaunt, had lost all his muscle mass, and even the muscles in his face had atrophied. Sometimes with AIDS, there can be a specific look on a person's face long before he dies. We had all come to recognize it and called it "the look of death." We saw it on Robert's face. We never told him what we suspected as we believed that he did not see it on his own face. Towards the end he asked me if he had "the look of death." I was startled and didn't know how to answer. I tried to muster a straight face and lie. I hoped lying would keep his spirits up. He responded by telling me that after seventeen years of friendship, he knew I was lying. I realized he had already surrendered his battle.

Later that November, Tony and I visited

him in the hospital. Robert had barely moved for hours, and it became time for me to drive Tony home. I wrote a letter to Robert because I was afraid he might die without me at his side. I left it in his hand and told the nurses to read it to him if he woke up. Here is what I wrote:

Dearest Robert,

Tony and I have been at your side for the past six hours and you have not made a sound. Tony has to work tomorrow so I am taking him home. If you should wake and I am not here, I am leaving you this note. You told me you are ready to go. I do not want you to give up. Please do not give up. I am worried that I may not be with you if you die. If that is the case, this letter may have to do.

Robert, you have been my best friend for seventeen years. I hold our memories in my heart. The best gift you gave me, other than your friendship, was helping me rejoin the living when I was the one too sick to get out of bed. I know you have suffered. I know you want to finally be in peace and comfort! Just the thought of not having you here leaves my heart hollow and my spirit broken. Right now tears are pouring down my face. I will be angry you are not going to be here to fight this dreadful disease with me. I will be disappointed to think you won't be here with me to celebrate a cure. Somewhere deep inside, I will be happy you are finally out of the pain and suffering. I will always miss you.

Your friend forever,

Joel

Robert died shortly after we left. He never got to hear my note, so I thanked God that I had already told him how much I cherished him.

That night made me think of my own life. Why am I still here? How long will I stay here? What will my last day on earth be like? With whom will I share it? I figured that since I can't know when that day will come, my best option is to treat every day as if it is my last. I realized that I was on a journey, and that it's not the destination that counts, it's the journey. I realized I could only find meaning in this moment of life because there might not be a next moment, a tomorrow, or a next year. Now is the time for living life to its absolute, fullest potential. That is how Robert's death changed my life.

I deeply missed Robert and felt sad after he died. However, the precious friendship that I created with him opened a place in my heart that never closed, even after his death. Losing my best friend did not shut down my soul. In time it had the opposite effect and allowed me to share love again. This kind of experience is invaluable for opening our hearts. We can cultivate the loving space in our core by manifesting it in our actions towards others. Trusting and loving have the great reward of bringing us more love. By sharing these qualities we will find ourselves surrounded by what we have given away. Giving unconditional love is magnetic. The more you give the more you receive. The place in my heart that had already been cultivated by a loving and trusting relationship was, in due time, ready to experience future wonderful relationships.

Robert's death was the first time I lost someone so close to me. He had been my ally for more than half my life. We had experienced most of our lives together, and now he was gone. Mark, Kelly, and Tony sensed the depth of my loss and went out of their way to support me.

The four of us would still go out to the movies or gather for a game of cards. We continued to get together for dinner at my place once a week, and we still had our deep conversations. We often felt that Robert was still with us.

Even in death there is no separation from those we love. Love is stronger than death.

Love transcends physical separation. We are connected by our love. Yet, at times the pain of loss can be searing, and that's because we feel separated. We are human and we hurt. Even if we forget for a time, we will ultimately remember the interconnectedness of our love. Viktor Frankl puts it this way "Love goes very far beyond the physical person of the beloved. It finds its deepest meaning in his spiritual being, his inner self. Whether or not he is actually present, whether or not he is still alive at all, ceases somehow to be of importance."

We are forever changed by those we love. Unconditional love is endless. We honor those who have died by continuing to live, in that they live on through our actions, our spirit, and our love. They become a part of us. They are a part of what we live and breathe, a part of our hearts. It's not just the memories that live on; the spark of the love that connects us never ends. That connection becomes a source of comfort and a warm glow. Love is truly eternal.

Chapter 4

Summer 1990–March 1994

"Every man can take the limit of his own field of vision for the limits of the world."

—Arthur Schopenhauer

A chance meeting in 1990 would change the entire course of my life. That summer, I ran into an old friend of Robert's and mine, named Albert Fleites. He had been living in Los Angeles for a few years. Robert and I had originally met him in Miami in 1974 when we were in high school. He was to become the most important friend of my life. I cannot explain why our friendship evolved to such a profound level. But, I am sure that chemistry, timing, and destiny played some role in it. If there is such a thing as a soul mate, he was mine.

When I reconnected with Albert, he was HIV positive. Yet, he was in perfect health. Albert too had lost his best friend to AIDS. We were both living amid the same holocaust. We each were grateful to have found someone else who had lived through the trials of youth return to confront the hardships of a life with AIDS. It was an immediate and strong bond that fueled the growth of a deep friendship. We needed each other in those days of great loss. The connection from our adolescence solidified our relationship. We shared joy, having known each other years before. Soon, we were seeing each other daily and the intertwining of our lives became more intense as time passed. Eventually, we understood each other without speaking words. Even at the most horrific times, we could lift each other's moods.

We did volunteer work at AIDS hospices. Supporting others took us out of our own distress. Together we searched for meaning in our lives. We also did typical things like going to the movies. More often than not our conversations were long and deep. At night we would often read to each other and explore theories about the afterlife. Albert had been intensely spiritual all of his life. He was a vegetarian, believing that all animals had souls. He was the gentle and sensitive soul, while I was the ambitious and practical one. In prior years, I had been a card-carrying member of The National Atheist's Association.

Our spiritual searching transformed me from complete atheist to a hopeful, yet skeptical, agnostic.

I introduced Albert to Tony, Kelly, and Mark, and they willingly adopted Albert into our small family. During the next four years, the five of us intensely valued our unconditional friendships and love. Self-expression seemed vital to each of us. Together, we were able to express our sadness, anger, and any other feelings that required an outlet. We knew that open and honest communication is vital for relationships to grow and prosper. We supported each other without any expectations, and we received tremendous joy in return. I discovered a type of direct cause and effect that is amazing; if love is what you give, then love is what you will get back. Even at this time of mortal danger I blossomed emotionally and had deeply loving experiences. If love could flower under these circumstances, it can flourish anywhere.

I made a concentrated effort to listen to my friends when they would open up. Relationships require empathy so we can understand and accept another person's position. Empathy is at the core of unconditional love. It is also key to a healthy, loving relationship. You can allow yourself to see those things you don't like in someone and then embrace them as a part of their uniqueness. By accepting their imperfections, we bring our relationships to a higher level.

Once again I'm talking about mastering the internal dialogue. People who impose conditions on their love usually transfer those conditions to themselves. People who accept other people's imperfections embrace their own humanness. We all have the capacity for unconditional love. Before we can share it with anyone else, though, we need to give it to ourselves. When you have negotiated within yourself to love unconditionally, you have made the choice to accept life on its own terms. Once you have made that choice, then you express a radiant joyousness without words to the people around you. You just exude love.

Sadly, during the next few years, the health of Mark, Kelly, and Tony rapidly declined. My health seemed to be improving. It seemed one of my friends was always ill or in the hospital. Among the things they faced: Tony had multiple lung infections, Mark was constantly being plagued with stomach infections, and Kelly had developed Kaposi's sarcoma cancer in his mouth. We were aware of the realistic possibility of developing opportunistic infections that we did not want to endure. We saw horrible suffering amongst those in the final stages of AIDS. We were all particularly afraid of blindness, of losing our mental faculties, or of having a tortured death.

Albert purchased the book *Final Exit* that explained how to commit suicide. Mark left the room when Albert shared the methods the book described, and he refused to take part in any such discussion. Tony, Kelly, and I were interested and read the book. It explained that a peaceful suicide required a large amount of narcotic sleeping pills taken very rapidly. The four of us decided to purchase enough drugs to kill ourselves. That way, if circumstances became too unbearable we could die peacefully rather than endure the agony AIDS might bring to our bodies. Kelly, Tony, Albert, and I made a promise that we would support whomever decided to end his own life. It wasn't death that I feared. I just wanted to die with some amount of dignity.

That winter, we each asked our doctors for a small amount of the narcotic. We planned to slowly stockpile the effective dose and not alert our physicians' suspicions. To our dismay, our doctors would not give us any of the drug. Our only choice was to buy it out of the country. Tijuana, in Mexico, was the most accessible place to acquire the illegal drug. Tony had the name of a Mexican pharmacy that would be accommodating. Tony got the name from a neighbor whose lover took his own life when he could no longer bear life with AIDS. So together we made the trip.

In Tijuana, we were instructed by the pharmacist to go to a small clinic and get prescriptions for the sleeping pills. The clinic was in a run down building that looked as if it had been neglected for a hundred years. It almost made 5p21 look clean. The difference was that at this clinic there were no other AIDS patients. The waiting room was filled with drug addicts waiting to get prescriptions for their drugs. The doctor saw us each separately and simply asked if we were having problems sleeping or dieting. Depending on your answer you would either get a prescription for narcotics or stimulants. I told him I was having problems sleeping. He asked me what dose and how many pills I needed. It was as simple as telling him exactly what I wanted to obtain. Before he gave me the prescription he demanded payment for the visit, which was one hundred and fifty dollars U.S. Each of us spent less then five minutes with the Mexican physician and obtained a prescription for the full lethal dose. We returned to the pharmacy and each bought one hundred Seconal pills.

We were extremely afraid to bring the drugs

back into the U.S. and did not want to get arrested. We were told of two ways to smuggle the drugs past the border patrol. We needed to either tape the bottles of pills to our bodies or ingest the pills in a condom. Each option had its advantage and disadvantage. Ingestion made them almost impossible to detect. Yet, ingestion had the risk that if the condom broke and we absorbed the drugs, we would die. That kind of death was scary, because at that point we were not ready to die.

Tony and I decided to tape ours to our legs. Kelly and Albert opted to ingest them. We held our breath driving through customs. But we weren't stopped, and my car was not even inspected. The officer simply waved us through the inspection lane. We all felt a sense of relief having obtained the drugs. We felt as if we finally had some control over our future.

By 1994, the health of Mark, Kelly, and Tony had so badly declined that Albert and I spent countless hours tending to their medical needs. I could not have done it alone. I remember a night in March when Mark called me at 3 A.M. He was running a high fever and was having trouble breathing. His health had been deteriorating the fastest of us all. It seemed as though Mark already had been through every opportunistic infection imaginable. This time, Albert and I rushed to his apartment and found him unconscious on his bathroom floor.

We carried his hot, wet, limp body to my car and drove him to the hospital emergency room. We learned his fever was over 104 degrees. The doctors told us he had yet another untreatable and potentially lethal lung infection. Mark had had zero T-cells for years which meant he had no functioning immune system at all. It was a wonder that he was still alive. Albert and I spent forty-eight hours by his bedside in constant vigil. We rubbed his body with ice in an attempt to make him comfortable any way we could. The doctors and nurses were waiting for him to die, and could not fathom that he would live. We, however, were not willing to underestimate Mark's strong desire to survive. To his physician's complete amazement, in less than a week, Mark pulled through. Somehow, remarkably, he had bounced back. Always the optimist, in just a matter of weeks, he was his old jovial self again.

During February and March, Albert and I spent nights at the bedside of either Mark, Tony, or Kelly. Tony and Kelly had become sick and one of them always needed care. It was during our time spent tending to the others that

Albert and I had our most serious conversations. Albert was devouring every book he could find on the subject of life after life. Despite my skepticism, I hoped for the possibility of life after death.

One night, Albert came up with the concept that whoever died first should try and signal the other from the beyond. It seemed like a good idea, and we promised to try to give the other an assurance of life after death. Even though I was a skeptic I was intent on keeping my vow to Albert. I loved him very deeply, and he was like a younger brother to me. I always felt protective towards him. It seemed reasonable to me that if there was an omnipotent God, and if I died before Albert did, God might do the favor of allowing me to signal him. If there was any possibility that I could signal, I would.

As the oldest and more sickly of the two of us, I figured I would die long before Albert. I was willing to attempt to barter my soul with God for a chance to signal Albert. After all, he was one of the kindest people I'd ever met, and surely God would allow me to impart some faith to Albert by this gesture. Albert would often remind me of our oath as if to check if I was still intent on keeping my promise.

Soon Kelly's Kaposi's sarcoma spread

throughout his entire body and he was beginning to show signs of dementia. At times he was delusional, and his conversations made little sense. This was horrible to watch, and we felt helpless. It was becoming a rare occasion when the five of us were able to get together as a group. Tony was so thin and fragile that he often refused to show up for our now infrequent dinners. This period marked the beginning of the end of our gatherings, and my friends' slow march into death. Instead of cooking on Thursday nights, I starting spending more time alone with Tony in his condo. He was getting ready to die. He was experiencing a kind of emotional death by becoming more withdrawn and shutting down his emotions. He was actually looking forward to the prospect of passing on. I was afraid he would take his own life. He was concerned that he would die and simply be forgotten. He often pleaded with me never to forget him. Somehow, he predicted that I would survive. He said, "You and Albert will be the two of us who live to see the cure. You both have a responsibility to remember those of us who die. You must never give up and keep fighting." He called me a brave soldier.

While all this sickness was going on, Albert and I became even closer. We continued to share our deep conversations daily and somehow, we were still able to laugh. It was during those months that we shared the most wonderful and joyous moments together. At that time, even meager pleasures provided us with intense happiness. Together, Albert and I always found freedom from the suffering.

One day in February, the five of us met for coffee at a cafe. We shared a wonderful time, and smiled and laughed for almost four hours. At one point, I left the table, and an acquaintance of Tony's stopped me to extend his sympathy towards Tony, Kelly, and Mark. He said, "It's so terrible what they are going through. They look so awful, I'm so sorry." Confused, I asked "Why?"

We were all very happy that afternoon. We were so joyous that we had forgotten about AIDS. His comments felt foreign compared to what we were experiencing. This man was focusing on physical deterioration rather than the joy and happiness that exuded from our table. His comments reflected his own fears rather than an accurate reflection of our moment. I was so absorbed in our joy that I actually didn't understand why he was extending sympathy. We both interpreted the same event differently. I saw an exuberant gathering of friends. He only saw the negative, a group of sick men.

In March of 1994, I started to get dark purple spots on my arm, then I got two of them on my face. During the past few years, I had changed doctors three times. I had decided not to continue seeing Dr. Roth because of his narrow vision about my survival, then my second doctor died of AIDS. I was being treated at this time by Dr. Robert Jenkins, who was Mark's doctor. I went in to see him, and we did a biopsy. Like Kelly, I had Kaposi's sarcoma and had to begin chemotherapy.

Similar to Dr. Roth eight years earlier, Dr. Jenkins predicted my life expectancy to be less than two years. But this time I was not devastated and released myself from his negative prediction. I knew he was wrong. It was that simple. I had learned to stay in the moment. I knew not to sabotage my chance of survival by worrying. However, it was a challenge to deal with an opportunistic infection that was visible in public.

When I first found out I had AIDS, vanity became a trivial concern. The bigger issue of survival took precedence over appearances. The dark purple cancer on my face was disfiguring, and common on people with advanced AIDS. It upset me because it created strong reactions in people, and I lost a sense of privacy. I could not hide the fact that I had advanced AIDS, and I disliked people looking at my face. Some people reacted with genuine concern while others shunned me.

During the first weeks of having this cancer on my face I had to muster courage to go out in public. In time, I adjusted and took people's reactions in stride. This cancer was yet another test of my determination. I was determined not to let it stop me from living. I went on about my life as if nothing had changed. The thing that hindered my functioning the most was the chemotherapy. It made me feel worn out and in pain. I was often doubled over a toilet vomiting. I fought like hell to get better.

Yet, within a month I was used to the fatigue and side effects from the chemotherapy. During the last two weeks in May, I decided to travel east to spend time with friends and family. After Robert died, I became keenly aware of the value of sharing time with those I loved. I vowed that the sarcoma was not going to stop me.

Chapter 5

June 1, 1994:

My Second Long Night—Acceptance

**"There are only two ways to live your life.
One is as though nothing is a miracle.
The other is as though everything is."**

—Albert Einstein

I was scheduled to return to Los Angeles on June 4, 1994. However, I was fatigued, so I decided to cut my trip short. I flew home on the morning of June 1. While I was away, I spoke with Albert almost every day. He seemed to be in good spirits. I was excited to see Albert and rushed home to surprise him.

I arrived at the house at noon. The bedroom was filled with spent candles. An empty wine bottle sat on the table, all the shades were drawn and the floor was strewn with empty capsules from the pills that we had gotten in Mexico. My friend, my family, my life, my joy had taken his own life. I went into shock and wept uncontrollably as I shook his cold gray body. I felt sick. My heart raced and my ears rang. I began wailing and screaming. Tears streaming down my face, I held and rocked his body. I felt like a lost child. He had taken his life and broken our promise. I was angry and convulsing. Neighbors heard my cries and called the police. They arrived and called the coroner. Why had he betrayed me? I needed an explanation, and I needed it immediately. Frantically, I searched the house for a note. It was what I needed more than anything else. I needed to know that Albert loved me, and that I was in his final thoughts. There was no note to be found.

I continued screaming and crying. I did not know how I would make it though the next hour, let alone the entire night. My heart was hollow, and for the first time in my life I felt totally alone and abandoned. I wanted to run, but there was no place to go. He had betrayed me at the very time I needed him the most. How shallow his love must have been. Every good thing we ever shared was meaningless. If he could do this to me, he must have never cared about me. I was so angry I shook, then hit his corpse.

His suicide was unexpected and triggered an avalanche of pain and anger. I couldn't care less about our pact to signal each other from the Beyond. If he wrote my name across the sky with a rainbow, I wouldn't care. Whatever he did wouldn't be as real as flesh and blood and friendship. He had abandoned me. I could hardly believe my best friend was gone, and by his own hand. I sat in despair for an unknown amount of time. The noise of people outside calmed down, and for a brief moment in the madness, I felt an eerie calm. It was as if I could feel his presence, as if he was actually talking to me. I did not hear words with my ears, but I sensed his faint cry.

I sensed that Albert was instructing me. He was telling me to go outside behind the house next door. There I would find a note in the trash. I followed his directions and found his last written words buried under garbage. It was the rough draft of a note that would arrive in the mail on June 4, my expected day of arrival. It allowed me to have some understanding of his motives and to know I was in his final thoughts and that he did love me. That was exactly what I needed to know, that I was indeed in his final thoughts. Its contents would haunt me for years, and not until I wrote this book have I been prepared to share it. I felt less betrayed, and that note carried me home.

To my most dearest love Joel,

By the time you get this note I will be dead. Writing this is the hardest thing I've ever had to do and I've been at it for five hours. The words won't come. The past few years have been both the most joyful and the most painful times of my life. It has truly been the best of times and the worst of times. I have cherished every single moment that we have been together.

All this love and doom is still everywhere I look. Death is on every corner of every street that I turn. It's on the faces of Kelly, Mark, and Tony, and now I fear it will soon be on yours. Someday it will be on mine, and I don't ever want you to see it on my face. The moment I heard Dr. Jenkins' words, everything changed. I realized I will someday lose you. That day would come as surely as it has for so many others. We both know this virus is relentless. I can not stand to watch you die or suffer. You are the stronger one of us, and you can handle life without me. I cannot go on and have wanted this since that moment Dr. Jenkins said the words Kaposi's sarcoma.

I am tired of watching everyone I love destroyed by this virus. I am too weak to go on. I pray you will find it in your heart to forgive me for doing it this way. I beg you to keep me in your heart. Perhaps in the next life I can be there for you as you were for me in this one. Try and be happy, understanding I am finally out of all the pain that has marked our lives. My final thought as I lay my head down will be of the smile on your face. I hope someday you will remember all the smiles we shared and not my death. Please don't ever forget me.

I will always LOVE you,

 Albert

Later that night, Albert came to me again, and then again in the days and months that followed. Time after time, I have pondered those ethereal moments. Despite living through those events firsthand, I still questioned them. I am a skeptic by nature and so are most of the people I have known. It's sensible to be one. You too may question Albert's ability to have signaled me from Beyond. It seems reasonable to believe that when a body dies, it is the end of life as we know it. It would be logical to assume that I simply thought that he put the draft in the trash and that I did not hear his psychic plea. You may think I imagined his voice or fabricated the story. I know I did not. Imaginary or not, those messages and events beginning the night he died would enrich and change the course of my life. I experienced a profound spiritual awakening. It doesn't really matter how I got this message. Regardless of its origin, its meaning is still the same. I cannot now tell you all the wondrous occurrences that transpired after his death. I've already written a book on just that. However, I can tell you the shimmering core of my epiphany.

Albert's core message to me was that each and every single moment of life has meaning and matters. Each moment of life is connected to something far greater than we can possibly see from our earthly perspective. Nor can we ever fully understand the purpose in every moment of our life. Even moments of pain and suffering have profound meaning and purpose. It was then I began to realize that every single second of life matters. In every moment, whether we know it or not, whether or not we can feel it, even during the most painful of moments, there is always a purpose. We cannot always feel it, but it exists nonetheless.

Let me use an analogy to explain Albert's message. Imagine that each second of your life is a droplet of water dripping from a faucet. Drop by drop they flow continually. You make this flow happen just by living. At the end of a day you have filled a glass of water; at the end of a week a bottle. The months fill a basin, the years begin to fill a pond. By the end of your life, you have filled an ocean. That volume of water marks the time we have spent on this planet. In that context, each individual droplet is a part of the whole body of water. Similarly, every second of every day is a significant component of your life.

Yet, every moment of life is even more miraculous from a divine viewpoint. Albert opened a window for me to peer through. I gained an elevated perspective on life. It was as if I was allowed to look into a microscope and examine a single "droplet" of my life. From that perspective I gained a deeper respect for the significance of each moment.

Under magnification a single droplet of water is teeming with life. If we were to examine a droplet of sea water under an electron microscope, we would see molecular universes that defy our comprehension. Simply by breathing and existing we are co-creating the universe of life that exists in each droplet. Each and every person is a vital part of the whole. Both cruel and kind people serve a purpose that we can't always understand. Even suffering is connected to a greater good. In every breath, we are working things out that we will never understand from our human perspective.

I gained a profound sense of faith from my

esoteric experiences that followed Albert's death. I came to believe all pain, loss, and suffering serves a greater good even if we can't see it in this lifetime. That faith gives me comfort. My suffering had meaning and purpose, even if I cannot understand it. In a way this book proves that to be true. If I am able to help even one person with my story, then my suffering has meaning. I still experience moments of physical pain, yet they are much easier to endure because I know they are a part of something greater.

I believe we are working things out in every moment of life. Life doesn't always feel good, and in fact, there are moments of great pain. Nonetheless those moments have meaning and purpose. It's much easier for me to go through the challenges of life with this belief than without it. My faith in this comforts me and has played a profound role in my healing.

Chapter 6

June 1994–December 1999
"Adversity introduces a man to himself."

—Anonymous

Life with AIDS was not the same as life without AIDS. I had to make major adjustments to survive. Paramount was accepting my condition and living in the moment. Living in the moment required me to accept new physical limitations. During the six months that followed Albert's death, my health steadily improved. I still had bouts with opportunistic infections, but I was getting stronger each week, even though I was helpless as the health of my three other friends worsened. Their deterioration could have made me afraid for my own health, but I clung to my optimism. It was an internal battle that I was determined to win.

Tony completely lost his will to live, and his

health steadily declined. He was constantly pessimistic and could not adjust to having AIDS. He was often stuck in anger. He resented AIDS for taking away his good looks and health. He could not find anything positive to focus on. Nothing I could say or do would pull him out of his despair. He was the next to die. He did not take his own life as I had suspected he would, but he died six months after Albert did. He simply gave up his will to live. His body just wasted away until he died. It was as if he willed death upon himself.

I found myself unable to care for Mark, whose health was also rapidly failing. Mark's loving family took him home to Denver to die, and he died several months later. He was the youngest of our group and had so much love for life. He was filled with plans until his last breath. Mark never believed he would die from AIDS. His strong will to live had kept him alive years beyond any medical expectation. Unlike Tony, he never gave up hope. Mark lived an extra decade with almost no functioning immune system, and that decade was filled with love, joy, life, and laughter. If the newer AIDS drugs had become available six months earlier, Mark would still be alive.

Later that year, Kelly's dementia worsened.

His conversations made little sense. I found it difficult to spend time with him. I was engaged in my own health battle with cancer, and we met only once a month for coffee. One of the last times we spoke, he informed me of the "cure" for Kaposi's sarcoma. He explained, "It's easy to use your fingernails and pick out the lesions by their roots, just like you would a weed." He showed me his method of removing the skin cancer by twisting his skin and subcutaneously poking his nails into it. Then he said, "See, I can just dig out the cancer."

I was horrified when he showed me his legs and arms. They were covered with open sores where he had been picking at himself to "cure" his cancer. I felt helpless and didn't know what to say. Instinctively I knew not to disagree with him or attempt to be rational. At a loss for words I responded with a forced smile that did not reflect my sadness. I strained and said, "Gee, Kelly that's great. Soon you'll be all better." The inability to engage in meaningful conversations with my last living friend caused even more grief. He was alive, yet he was not with me. We slowly lost touch. A relative of Kelly's called me to tell me he died in 1996.

On that day, I pulled out my phone book from my dresser drawer. One by one, I turned to the pages that had held Kelly, Mark, and Tony's names, addresses, old phone numbers, and vital information. I wrote "dead" in red ink over and over across the page. I stopped when the pen pierced through the paper, and I could no longer read their names. All that was left on those pages was red ink.

Tony, Kelly, and Mark were all younger than me. In just a matter of months I had watched them deteriorate. Before my eyes, they went from robust young men in their prime to frail, sickly, gray, dying men. This was the end of my family. I was now alone.

I had no place to look for support except within myself. Again, I would have to reach into my core to find the courage to continue. I would force myself to continue living. Albert's message of hope and purpose was a blessing at that time. Underneath all my grief, I felt blessed to have shared deep loving relationships for several wonderful and amazing years. I had been friends with Tony, Kelly, Mark, and Albert for years, yet in the grand scheme of things it was a blink of an eye. Somehow I felt they were still with me and that I would see them again. The time we spent together had been a journey that I would not change for all the money in the world. I was blessed to have had them in my life.

I used the same slow, methodical pace to heal from the Kaposi's sarcoma as I did from my first lung infection. I survived the bad days by focusing on any good moment they contained. An open window with a pleasant breeze, sunshine, seeing the trees outside all meant so much to me. Each hour without pain revitalized my spirit.

For the most part, my body was responding well to the chemotherapy, although it repressed my red and white blood cells as AZT did in 1987. New drugs to raise cell levels had been developed a few years earlier and my doctor was able to prevent any serious complications. In just a few months the cancer was in remission. Things got even easier in 1996 with the advent of the new AIDS drugs called protease inhibitors. My health rapidly improved after taking them. I regained my physical strength and was able to return to my cardiovascular fitness training.

As my health was improving, I realized that I had to deal with other aspects of living. Often, I was just going through the motions of living. One day I felt well driving in my car on my way to work out. I stopped at a red light, and noted the girl in the car next to me was singing out loud to the music on her radio. She looked happy and smiled at me. I wanted to be happy. Her radio was tuned to the same station as mine. "Baby Love" by the Supremes was playing. I loved old Motown songs, and that song had been one of my favorites. In that moment, hearing a song that used to bring me joy, I realized I now felt none. For a few moments, I was jealous of the other motorist and her carefree happiness. I resented her happiness. I wanted to sing in my car again. I wanted to dance in my car. I wanted to feel joy, but I was flat.

At the next red light I looked in the mirror and saw my reflection. I looked solemn. I looked at my clothing and saw that everything I had on was old. I had not been shopping for new clothes in years. I had stopped going to the movies or out to dinner. While driving, I had been eating a candy bar for energy and noticed that I had not enjoyed its sweetness. It was a beautiful day and I hadn't noticed that. My health was okay that day, and I was on my way to work out, but I wasn't happy. Later, during my exercising, I realized I was just going through the motions and was not challenging my body. I found myself in an emotional purgatory.

I had survivor's guilt, and it was numbing me, keeping me from the life before me. Kelly, Mark, Robert, Albert, and Tony would have wanted me to continue my fight and so I did. I needed to rejoin the living if I was to survive. But, I had become afraid to make new friends, because I was petrified of further loss. However, I forced myself to try, and hesitantly, I began to make plans to do things with people. I invited neighbors to dinner or the theater and began to make new friendships.

It was an uphill road to rejoin the living. I had to reteach myself to experience joy. It was just like taking small steps towards physical healing. I took small steps towards emotional healing. I started by renting funny movies and doing things that I used to enjoy. I began to work in my garden again and to take walks. I forced myself to look on the bright side. I was not the same person as I was before AIDS. I was more thoughtful and had respect for each moment of life.

As time progressed, my sadness lessened. The passing of time is an amazing thing: plants grow and blossom; friendships deepen; grief softens. After a few months, I could go weeks without feeling sad. I was returning to normalcy. In time, I was able to laugh and smile again.

There was no magical technique to survive AIDS and loss. My transformation from sickness to physical health took time and so did my emotional healing. Survival became a lifetime commitment. Living in the moment was key to reducing fear and staying strong. I made lifestyle changes that began with acceptance and moved on to making choices to facilitate better health. I cannot overemphasize the importance of acceptance, living in the present, and a willingness to adjust to life's new terms. With acceptance you can begin to see disease or any challenge as part of your whole life experience. Embracing suffering as part of the whole can help you transcend any obstacle. Pain and suffering do not feel good, and it is natural not to want to feel them. My faith is that every moment of life has meaning and purpose. The purpose of suffering is often beyond my comprehension. Even though some moments of life don't feel good, they still have meaning. Knowing that my suffering is not just in vain and is connected to something greater has given me faith to stay in the present moment with acceptance.

One evening in March 1996, I invited a neighbor to see a comedy. I hoped to distract myself from the pain of an intestinal infection I was fighting. While driving to see the movie, I had diarrhea in my clothes. I was frustrated, humiliated, and disgusted. I was mad that we missed the movie because I had to go home to shower off. In a rare moment of anger, I yelled out, "Why me, Lord? Haven't I suffered enough? God, could you just give me a break?"

I was still mad even after cleaning up. Once I was changed, we decided to drive and get some soup and a baked potato. While I was eating my soup, a quadriplegic entered the restaurant. He had movement only in one hand and part of his face. He had a nurse to spoon-feed him. All of his body, even his face, was atrophied. His electric wheel chair was covered with bumper stickers and slogans: Greenpeace, Amnesty International, and stickers about kindness. I thought to myself, "Who am I to complain? At least I am able to drive home and take a hot shower. At least I'm able to walk into a restaurant and feed myself."

My focus shifted back to him. It was wonderful to see someone in that condition still getting out, still obviously involved in life. When we went to exit the restaurant I smiled at him. He smiled back and said in a quiet voice "Oh my God, Joel, how are you? I haven't seen you in ten years or more." I didn't recognize him. He continued, "Well I'm so glad you are OK. When I don't see someone for awhile who I know has AIDS I tend to worry if they are still alive. You look well. Do you know my story?"

I looked into his eyes and answered, "No, but I think it's great that you are getting out and about."

Just as the words came out of my mouth, something in his eyes became familiar and I realized who he was. Richard had been a gregarious, handsome, athletic friend of Tony's. When I realized how much he had deteriorated, I could not hold back my tears. As soon as he saw me cry, he snapped back, "Please don't cry for me. I have the greatest life; let me tell you about it. Several years ago I was training for the California AIDS ride from Los Angeles to San Francisco. I was riding my bike on Coldwater Canyon and was hit by a car that broke my neck. After the accident, I lay for weeks in Cedars-Sinai hospital in a deep depression. On my third week, a high school football player was brought in with a broken back from a sports injury. The kid was so angry that he was cursing everyone and begging the nurses to kill him.

"When I heard his yelling and screaming, I had an epiphany. I decided I would go back to UCLA and get my Ph. D. in psychotherapy so I could counsel people who have life-altering injuries. I was lucky and got the first job I applied for. It's at Cedars, and I am now doing exactly what I love to do. I'm helping people like me every day. Isn't that great?"

He was filled with joy, satisfaction, and happiness. I was shocked to see such joy and pride light up his face. As I stood in the presence of his resilient and joyous spirit, I felt humbled. He had been reborn through his suffering. Here was a hero who had risen to the occasion of his life. When he had gone back to school he didn't have the benefit of two working hands to type, so he had to wear special glasses that shot a laser beam at an adapted computer screen. He typed one letter at a time by blinking one eye and triggering the laser beam mechanism. His Ph. D. took fifty times the effort of an average unimpaired doctoral candidate but he still achieved it in half the time. I was speechless.

"WOW!" was all I could say as I thought about his life. He made the choice to go through it with dignity and grace and to rise to a level higher than his suffering. He was living in the now and there he found joy.

I compared my situation to that which he suffered as a quadriplegic and felt gratitude. I focused on things I had in my life, rather than my problems. I had use of my arms and legs. I had a comfortable place to live and good medical care. I even had new friends. My life was enriched when I encountered Richard in his wheelchair, and I became even more grateful for each moment of life. His life is a shining example of hope, acceptance, and of embracing life.

Chapter 7

December 28, 1999:

A Third Long Night—Emotions

**"There is a very fine line between triumph
and disaster. That line is hope."**

—Joel Rothschild

By December of 1996, I was coping well
with AIDS despite still having short bouts with
opportunistic infections. The two worst of these
were ongoing neuropathy and reoccurring herpes
zoster, both of which affect nerves and result in
pain. Yet, I had learned to transcend physical
pain. Somehow, the more I lived through, the
more I could handle. A side effect from the new
medicines was fatigue. I simply slowed down the
pace of my life to accommodate the fatigue. To
someone unfamiliar with physical pain, my average day might feel like having a bad flu. After ten
years of living with AIDS, I had become a
stronger person. I constantly would remind
myself that even the painful moments of life

have deep meaning and purpose and that it's OK not to see it. I took myself to a place of acceptance. I was learning to embrace all of life, not just the moments that felt good.

I never gave into the fear created by Dr. Jenkins' words that I would die from the cancer. If I had surrendered to his prognosis, I would have been giving away the right to live my life on my terms. Instead, I stepped through my fears and believed I could handle whatever happened medically. After all, I had already outlived Dr. Roth's prediction of my death by over a decade and I was in my bonus round. In spite of AIDS, I was a happy person. I was grateful for life. I had made several new friends and I had even fallen in love with a scientist named Dr. Keith Del Villar, Ph.D. I had achieved a level of happiness and serenity that previously seemed impossible to me. I had been blessed in many ways.

It may be hard to believe, but I know that in the end, all of the suffering that we experience ultimately enriches our lives and strengthens our spirit. The period between 1996 and 1999 with Keith was a time of great healing. As each month passed, I had regained more strength.

On December 28, 1999, I had reason to

celebrate. My viral load was nearly unde-
tectable and my T-cell count was almost normal. I had been in a relationship with Keith for
almost three years, and I cherished it. I found
love again, something I previously thought was
reserved for only those who had the time to
grow old together and explore life with another
soul. I was excited about life's prospects in the
new millennium.

That December day, I had come home early
to plan a New Year's surprise for Keith. Oddly, I
found him at home packing his clothing. He
began to tell me that he had met someone else,
fallen in love, and decided to leave me. He had
come home early to pack his clothing and was
leaving immediately to meet his new lover in
New York. I was in shock. The new abandonment
opened up memories of all my other losses.

That night as Keith walked out of my life, I
reeled into a downward emotional spiral. In an
instant, the glass was half-empty, not half-full.
Life seemed to be without hope. I began to
focus on the negative. I started to hate my life.
Every wound I'd ever experienced in life
seemed to re-open. It was like a sledgehammer
that smashed my heart. Even though I had survived the devastation of losing my closest
friends, this unexpected loss seemed more than

I could bear. The depression that ensued forced me to question my existence. It pitted logic and reason against raw emotion in a battle. With Keith's departure, my emotions shifted one hundred and eighty degrees in a flash.

I thought that many had died from a broken heart, and I started to understand how that could happen. I felt weak and afraid. The silence of the night seemed hostile. My existence seemed utterly meaningless. Why carry on with my continual struggle? What was the point in continuing to live? My heart felt wounded, and soon my immune system became affected. I quickly got the flu and developed an intense fever. Too embarrassed to call friends for help, I was in bad shape.

Even Billy, our Jack Russell terrier, seemed to lose his joy. For the next two days he would sit and wait by the front door for Keith to come home. He didn't even play with his favorite tennis ball, he moped around the house. Not once during those dreadful days did he wag his tail.

After seventy-two hours of not eating, not sleeping, and lots of crying and panic, I decided it was time to end our lives. I wanted out. At three A.M., December 30, 1999, I opened the bottle of little red Seconal capsules that Albert and I had gotten together in Mexico. I mixed them with yogurt. I took two Tigan left over from my chemotherapy to keep me from vomiting up the concoction. I saved ten Seconals for Billy and planned to put them into hamburger meat or force them down his throat after I ate half of my yogurt. I slowly began eating the bitter yogurt and washing down the taste with rum and Coke. With each spoonful, I was more steadfast in my resolve to end my life. But I was not eating the concoction quickly enough.

I started to feel sleepy and peaceful. I'm not sure if it was the effect of the drugs or exhaustion. At that moment, Billy became animated and did something he had never done before. One by one, he brought me all of his toys that were scattered around the house. His tail was wagging; he wanted to play. He tossed his tennis ball to me and began to bark. In his eyes I saw the love for life I could not feel. I stared at his joyous face. In his happiness, he was completely unaware of my pain. It became clear to me that I had no right to take his life, and I shouldn't take mine. I knew there was infinitely more to life than what I was now feeling.

Billy engaged me in a game of tug-of-war. He kept me awake for thirty-five minutes with his antics. I saw a glimmer of my own hope reflected in his playful joy. I did not finish the yogurt. I felt tired and eventually passed out.

I awoke about an hour later to Billy licking my face. I had always loved my little dog and now it seemed as if he was looking out for me. I began to think about the fun we had in the past playing Frisbee and taking long walks on our hillside together. Those simple happy memories shined a light on the part of me that loved life. I felt a spark of hope. I found myself once again questioning what I held dear, reaching inside for strength. Deep inside, I knew I would heal from this loss. I knew that even the most beautiful experiences come and go. Inside was an undercurrent of hope that I had gained from my years of living with AIDS. At times, the hope was so strong, it was almost palpable.

That night hope was in the distant background but moving towards me. I walked around my home. Tears came to my eyes, thinking I had almost killed myself. Billy was trailing behind me in a jovial prance. I marveled over his beauty and aliveness and the miracle that had unfolded. I broke out of my isolation, called two new friends and told them my situation. They both canceled their New Year's plans and rallied to my side and for the next three days were constantly with me. They were understanding and reinforced the thought that time heals all wounds, my pain would pass, and this was a temporary setback that I could handle. I was past my lowest moment. I knew I would feel joy and peace again.

When it came to love, I knew how much to give and when to walk away. I did not project my needs onto the relationship. I looked at the relationship as it really was and not as how I would have it be. I had long ago stopped trying to control people, situations, and outcomes. I knew just as people grow and change, so it is with love, and we don't have the right to demand love on our terms. I needed to let go.

A few weeks later while walking Billy I heard two elderly, wrinkled women complaining about life as they sat on a park bench. They were engaged in a conversation that resembled a fencing match. They exchanged words like weapons as they swapped "war" stories about their lives. At first they cursed their children. One said, "My children haven't visited me in over a month." The other would take a stab at minimizing her friend's issue by saying, "Well, my kids haven't called me in over three months and I've not spoken to my grandchildren in that whole time."

Each subject would regress to the lowest possible point, and then they would shift the conversation to another issue. The next round went like this; "Well, it's a good thing you don't have to see them often. Last month when I saw my daughter-in-law, it was horrible. All she did was complain about money." Her opponent responded, "Well, at least she was complaining about money. My son has been so sick with diabetes they thought he might have to go into the hospital."

The women shifted the conversation to another battleground. "Talking about health, I've been so sick with diabetes sometimes I can hardly walk, and my gout is killing me." The other interjected, "My sugar count is much worse than yours and the doctor says I'm at risk for blindness." The other then said, "Better to be blind than dead."

Their joyless conversation went on and on in this never ending cycle, each woman trying to win the argument by minimizing the other's feelings. The prize would be an acknowledgment that indeed her life was the more awful life.

Neither woman could focus on the fact that it was a gloriously beautiful day. Life on that day in the park was a bitter contest over the perceived miseries of existence. It made me think about how my own pain had kept me from feeling joy. After everything I'd been through, Keith's leaving was a small matter. It was time to forgive him and focus on the positive in my life.

Perhaps at times a comparison of someone else's suffering can help us to focus on our own situation with more clarity. However, our suffering is still ours, and we don't suffer equally. Think of the fable about the boy who was crying because he had no shoes until he saw someone with no legs. If you are crying because you have no shoes, you still ache that you have no shoes even if someone else has no legs. The suffering that is yours is real to you. It is worthy of your feelings.

So is the joy in recognizing that life itself is a gift. Suffering is something to learn from, process, and release. The person who has no legs may adapt better to his situation than the person who has no shoes. Those two women were focusing on what was "bad" in their lives, but I'm talking about making conscious choices to focus on the positive. I'm talking about learning to shift our perspective. You can make peace and joy constants in your life. Whether or not they are tangible in this moment of your life they are still attainable. It is possible to allow peace and bliss into your life despite your circumstances.

Life is given to us. Each moment of life is a gift for us to receive. Although we experience moments of pain, nonetheless, they too are a gift, an opportunity for change. We may not be happy about certain events in our lives but we can be thankful for the opportunity to do something about them. Within each moment is the chance to rejoice. We can find joy even in our most challenging moments. Joy is a kind of happiness that doesn't depend on what is happening. Normally, we are happy when things go our way and unhappy when something happens that we do not consider good. We can be joyous no matter what happens.

Happiness is linked to gratitude. We can be thankful for whatever is given to us, no matter how difficult. That is a choice we can all make. We can start by expressing gratitude for the things we usually take for granted. We have eyes to open and see beautiful things. We have ears to listen to sounds, legs to walk with, and lungs to breathe with. Are these things not worthy of our gratitude?

Chapter 8

Forgiveness and Love

**"The weak can never forgive.
Forgiveness is the attribute of the strong."**

—Mahatma Ghandi

Practicing forgiveness and love every day is the ultimate goal to which we can aspire. The act of forgiveness is clearly a choice. We make that choice for ourselves. It is our salvation. It is not a favor that we give to those who have wronged us. When we forgive, we choose to heal. When we have been hurt or wronged, we can hold on to the bad feelings, keeping them inside where they fester and poison our lives. By forgiving and letting go, we release the anger and hurt to our benefit.

For me, it was time for me to let go, to walk away and forgive. I needed to forgive Keith for leaving and myself for attempting suicide.

I began my emotional healing by forgiving

Keith for cheating on me. It would have been easy for me to fixate on Keith and my negative thoughts. So, I made a conscious choice to stay present with my feelings and forgive. This was a great healing force. It seemed like a light bulb went off. I remembered a voice in my head at 5p21; "This is it . . . You might have one year or one day, but it's definitely time to stop waiting for life to happen and to start living as if each day is your last." I did not want to squander my life by living under a cloud of impending doom. I knew that life is seldom fair, and we don't always get what we think we deserve. Sometimes, bad things do happen to unsuspecting good people. Often, that's just the way life goes.

I realized how blessed I was to have lived all those years since my time in 5p21. I knew that there is infinitely more to life than we realize. I began to feel the soothing calmness of gratitude. I felt at peace with the world. I felt appreciation for not killing myself. I felt a pure joy in just living. I understood the overwhelming power of forgiveness. It was then that perhaps I approached a state of enlightenment. The moment was not marked with a loud bang or even a quiet whimper. It was when the focus of my entire life was narrowed down to a single word: forgiveness. Forgiveness for myself and for everyone that I have ever, and will ever, encounter in this life.

When you make the choice to forgive, that will be the moment you, too, scratch the surface of the Divine. You will be choosing to step forward out of the jungle into the heights of humanity. You will stand side by side with God and all his genius. You will tap into and manifest the unlimited and eternal power of the Universe. All this, and you have only moved one inch beyond mediocrity and an ordinary existence.

After all, mediocrity is a self-inflicted condition, and this miracle a self-bestowed choice. Moving that one inch into the Divine allows us to experience an infinitesimal particle of the vastness of creation. That tiny particle is less than a teardrop in the ocean, a droplet that can positively transform all you have ever, and will ever, experience.

Making the choice to forgive can expand your sense of self. We must also forgive our perceived "failures." We do so by releasing events that don't go the way we expect. If you judge yourself in terms of your perceived failures or dashed expectations, that narrow frame of reference is only going to create more "failure." When you focus on limitations and failure you are looking at life from a very small perspective. In reality, life is so big it is impossible for us to comprehend the vastness and potential of what tomorrow will bring.

There is a simple law of nature that if things don't work out one way, another opportunity will always arise. If you don't reach a goal, that is the Universe saying to you "Make another goal, that's where your potential lies." Holding onto what you perceive as a failure will narrow your focus and cause you to miss life's next opportunity.

We all have the innate ability to almost instantaneously release negative thoughts, and see our positive potential. That internal processing of events, by focusing on the positive rather than the negative, is common amongst survivors and highly successful people. One of life's greatest lessons is to learn that we each have the ability to process, to release, and to move ever closer to expressing our inherent genius. That is true optimism. Choose to focus on your glass being half-full rather than half-empty, and the universe will replenish the entire glass.

If you hold on to your failures and beat yourself up about them, you will experience further negative spiraling. You sabotage yourself, and this sabotaging is rooted in any negative voices that you heard while growing up. You are governed by fear. When you hold on to your emotional frustration from unconsummated expectations, you resist the fullness of your potential. You are without acceptance. To release negativity, a key first step is to become aware of your own consciousness. You can't process or be liberated from what you're not aware of. All the therapy in the world is not going to help people who are not conscious about what they are doing to themselves.

I would probably be dead by now if I held on to events that did not go my way. When I first heard Dr.Roth's negative prognosis that I had less than a year to live, I was sent reeling into a panic attack. His words held power because they triggered my deepest fears. If I had allowed those words to penetrate my psyche and resonate there with their lethal message, I would have died, and done so in the grip of fear.

My choice to process and then release his negative comments was essential to my survival. It allowed me to consider the possibility of living instead of dying. I made the choice internally and it helped me stay alive. That tiny shift in thought is part of what kept me from joining the ranks of the twenty million AIDS victims. My belief that I would live proved to be more powerful than the negative spiral that I experienced as a result of his words.

For you now reading my words, here is a direct example of this lesson. Here is a healing gift you can give yourself. It is an offering from your last "failure" or an event in your life that did not go "your way." Consider an expectation of yours that was not fulfilled. Feel your anger or disappointment about what could have been. However, don't let it consume you. Remember, the negativity can poison you and limit your potential. Consider other grander possibilities and the vastness of your potential. Release your negative judgments and accept the reality of your present situation.

Now, try to let go of your unfulfilled expectation. In this very moment, you can experience the calming effect of acceptance and forgiveness. You have just walked yourself into the light. Welcome to the moment. You have just scratched the surface of the Divine.

Chapter 9

Spring 2000:

The Duality of Our Existence

"The unexamined life is not worth living."
—Socrates

Having the remarkable luxury to be able to look back, I'm amazed at the power of emotions. It was purely an emotional response that brought me to the brink of suicide. I was feeling pain that, intellectually, I knew would pass. Yet my intellectual understanding had little effect on the raw emotions. I was functioning on conflicting levels. I had the capacity to create more pain or to bring greater serenity into my life. I did not resist or numb my sadness. Doing so would only prolong the discomfort. I allowed myself to experience, and then process, my pain.

Pain and loss are a part of the human condition. In time we are often able to see benefits from suffering. Time alone often heals us and in adversity we can grow. When we are forced to face our fears we learn of our greatest strengths. Suffering strips away our illusions and humbles us. We often think that we are invincible and in control of our lives, but we are all going to suffer setbacks and pain.

A friend once said that the only way to get over pain is to go through it. You can't avoid or bypass it. She compared it to childbirth. Despite excruciating pain, the birth process can't be stopped in the middle. Yet out of that pain, a new life will enter this world. She was right, and during my healing process this book was born.

My experience with Keith enabled me to understand the duality of our existence. As human beings we are often pulled in conflicting directions. It is the nature of our existence to experience these polarities. On one end of the spectrum, the way we experience our existence is the result of living in the physical world and facing the challenges of satisfying our basic human needs. Functioning in the physical realm demands our almost constant attention. Our survival depends on it. We need to take care of basic physiological needs and then practice acceptance and forgiveness.

Yet, we are also spiritual beings and experience moments from the other end of the spectrum. Here we transcend our separateness and experience God within us. This is when you know your suffering has meaning and purpose. These are the moments of enlightenment. These are the moments, both big and small, that have inspired greatness. As we encounter these moments, we find ourselves connected to our higher self, to the Divine, to God and the Universe. It is perhaps the highest state we can achieve within our humanity. Part of our challenge is to figure out how to spend as much time as possible in this enlightened state of being, because it is from this state that we grow.

Experiencing these two states of being is like living in two different houses. In the house in which we begin our journey to enlightenment, we feel disconnected from each other and from God. All of our painful experiences and memories have built this house. I do not want to label this a bad place. For many people this house is a place of safety. However, the familiarity of this dark house can become a trap, causing us to live a fear-based life and to cower at what might lie outside. This is the house that contains hateful judgments against other people and ourselves. We are our own worst enemy in this house, and often we are not even aware of it. We can be lost in the dark with the blinds closed and the drapes drawn.

In this house, we can have a false sense of strength and never know our true capabilities. If we look inside, we believe ourselves to be weak, and these beliefs limit our potential. In this house, we feel despair and loneliness. In this house, the glass is always half-empty and the mirrors do not reflect our true selves or God within us. In this dark house, we are not going to survive any disease. Our chances of healing and surviving await us in the other house. We can try to catch ourselves when we are in the dark house. It has become a priority of mine in order for me to stay alive.

The other house is filled with love and kindness. Its foundation is rooted in our innate capacity to love. In this house we do not judge. We accept people as they are. We learn to accept other people's shortcomings and frailties, and in the process, peace and contentment are born of forgiveness. This forgiveness extends not only to other people, but to ourselves as well. We come to know that when we are pointing fingers at others, we are most likely judging ourselves. In this house, we hold our hopes and dreams. We are our own best friend. This house is composed of all the positive and affirming elements in our lives. We sense we are connected to each other and the universe. This house is filled with light and in it we know how strong we are.

We know we are larger than our bodies. It is here that we can come to realize the wondrous nature of our uniqueness and we embrace the entirety of who we are and what we have experienced. We are all actually a singular universe within ourselves, replete with living organisms and complete environments. Yet all of us are made of the same components. Our blood contains the minerals of the sea, and our flesh is made of the compounds of the Earth. If we look within, we can see our own bodies mimicking the very structure of nature. We can truly know that we are all connected and part of something greater. We are all assembled from the same core building blocks of life. We are all a part of God. Yet, we also have a profound effect on the whole of God. It is as if we are all individual grains of sand on a great beach, which is God. Our primary duty is to polish our individual grains so the beach glows with shimmering light.

Some of us have settled comfortably into

the dark house and others into the bright house. It is in our nature to move back and forth between the two houses. This transition occurs as a reaction to events in our lives. It is change that can create discomfort in either house.

The more serenity we experience in our lives, the greater our resilience to the negative effects of change. It will become less often that you find yourself back in the dark house. When you make the bright one your permanent residence, you will begin to recharge your energy and the energy of those around you. Our lives become miraculous and we can ease the transition of others. Soon we find ourselves living life with purpose and meaning. In this house, we can fulfill our destinies and achieve our dreams. In the house of light, we can discover the life we were born to live.

My thoughts of suicide are an example of when I ran out of the bright house back into the dark house. Immediately prior to that, I was soaring. It was the end of December of 1999, and I felt contented and blessed. Then everything abruptly changed. In January 2000, I was suicidal. I never thought I would experience a setback of that magnitude after all the challenges I had survived. But, as long as there is life, there are challenges we cannot avoid. It all comes back to making choices. When we feel as if we do not have a choice, we are in the dark house. We are trapped there and do not see what our choices are. We always have choices; we just don't allow ourselves to see them.

When I ran into the dark house, I was subliminally sabotaging myself, playing old well-acquainted tapes in my head. I was sending messages to myself like: "If I was better looking or if I didn't have AIDS, I would not be alone." My belief was that I was less than adequate. My thoughts were that nobody would ever love me again, that I was the ugliest person alive. In reality, Keith's leaving had nothing to do with me. His leaving had to do with his confronting *his* issues.

When we begin to recognize our emotional reactions to events, they become less turbulent. The strength I accrued surviving the difficult physical infections allowed me to move from the dark house back into the light house. Doing so, I realized the negative effects that self-sabotage could have on my physical health.

It remains a simple, universal fact that we will all be touched by loss and will inevitably suffer in the course of our lifetimes. At some point, we all experience changes that affect us physically and emotionally. The loss of dreams, aspirations, expectations, or relationships can shift our perspective. They are often life altering and can serve as catalysts for depression, angst, and fears. Even the anticipation of such changes can produce catastrophic consequences. We can internalize fears until they wreck our chances at happiness, or even kill us.

No one can live life one hundred percent of the time in a place of enlightenment. No matter how good we are at mastering life, it is going to deal us enough situations to send us emotionally reeling. When we experience these unforeseen setbacks, sometimes we have to start all over again, and that's okay. I had to start healing by forgiving myself for being human and allowing myself to experience my full range of emotions. Sometimes we just have to put one foot in front of the other and walk. Sometimes we have to force ourselves to meet the challenges of life. Sometimes it takes every ounce of strength and courage to do what's right for ourselves. Sometimes it's not easy to forgive but it's never impossible.

The one constant in life is that everything will change. Just around the corner can be a new and astounding experience. No matter who or where you are, you are capable of transforming your state of being. You can escape the enslavement of the dark house and enter the enlightened state of consciousness. You can even sustain it in your life. The choice is yours.

Chapter 10

March 14, 2001:

Conclusion

"Discovery consists not in seeking new landscapes, but in having new eyes."

—Marcel Proust

Today a friend who works at CNN called to tell me that life expectancies for people with AIDS have been increased. Then he faxed me excerpts from the following report.

AP 3/14/01 Atlanta

In a report today that cited five recent government studies, the U. S. Centers for Disease Control raised the median life expectancy of a person with full-blown AIDS living in the U. S. This is the first increase in over ten years. The CDC reports that in 2001 the median life expectancy of a person diagnosed with full-blown AIDS is now thirty-nine months. That figure is four times higher that the previous figure of eleven months in 1991.

I called my friend back and reminded him that I have been living with full-blown AIDS for more than fifteen years. He said, "That's how you have come to see the value of *each day* of life." I responded, "*each moment* of life."

I have now lived forty-four years on this planet. That is about twenty-three hundred weeks or sixteen thousand days. I have lived with full-blown AIDS for most of my adult life. When I was diagnosed there were less than thirty thousand cases globally and today there are more than thirty million. During my years of living with AIDS, we have lost twenty million people to this disease, and I have lost my five closest friends.

Now, I hug a little tighter and embrace people a few seconds longer. All of my memories are a little brighter and more meaningful. The colors of daylight are more brilliant and vivid. I am less fearful and the solutions to all of life's problems are more simple. Music sounds richer to my ears. My love is a little stronger and deeper. I cherish a smile on the face of a stranger as much as the memory of a smile on the faces of Robert, Tony, Kelly, Mark, or my beloved Albert. Billy's little wagging tale can bring a tear of joy to my eyes. These days, all people seem a little more beautiful.

When you get to that place of knowing that each and every moment of life matters, life becomes a peaceful and wondrous existence. You stop fighting the little battles and trust that all of life has a purpose. It becomes OK not to know what the purpose is. Somewhere deep inside, you know that your acts of kindness and love truly last forever.

About the Author

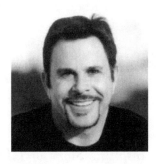

Joel Rothschild was born and raised in Miami Beach, Florida. He received his degree in communications from Florida Atlanta University in 1979. He was a competitive bodybuilder and owned a highly successful health spa before being diagnosed with full-blown AIDS on April 22, 1986. He has outlived more than twenty million people that have died from AIDS since that time. According to the U.S. Centers for Disease Control statistics, Joel Rothschild is one of the longest-living AIDS survivors in the world today.

He has volunteered, assisted, and worked with terminally ill people for more than eighteen years and has worked pro-bono as an AIDS activist and domestic lobbyist specializing in the Food and Drug Administration's new drug-testing policies. From 1987 to 1998 he served as a volunteer medical "guinea pig" and is the lone survivor from several FDA drug studies. He still actively volunteers and supports several charities. He has appeared on numerous national television and radio shows. On March 31, 2001, the National Academy of Television Arts and Sciences bestowed upon him one of their highest honors, the 2001 TV Cares Award. He is the author of the best-selling *Signals, An Inspiring Story of Life after Life*, currently published worldwide in nine languages. Joel lives in Los Angeles and shares his home with two Jack Russell terriers, Gertie and Billy. He is currently writing his third book, *Other People's Signals*.

Speaking Engagements

Joel Rothschild is available on a limited basis for speaking engagements and seminars. Every effort will be made to accommodate those that benefit charitable organizations.

To contact Mr. Rothschild, please write to: P.O. Box 38773, Los Angeles, CA 90038, or e-mail: abook4all@aol.com, or visit his website www.joelrothschild.com

Hampton Roads Publishing Company

. . . for the evolving human spirit

Hampton Roads Publishing Company
publishes books on a variety of subjects including
metaphysics, health, complementary medicine,
visionary fiction, and other related topics.

For a copy of our latest catalog,
call toll-free, 800-766-8009,
or send your name and address to:

Hampton Roads Publishing Company, Inc.
1125 Stoney Ridge Road
Charlottesville, VA 22902
e-mail: hrpc@hrpub.com
www.hrpub.com